MW00512564

Keto Diet Recipes

The Complete Cookbook to Success with
the Ketogenic Diet.
Delicious, Easy and Simple Low Carb
Recipes for Weight Loss, Reverse Diabetes
and Live Healthy.
The Keto Lifestyle Guide.

Alexangel Kitchen

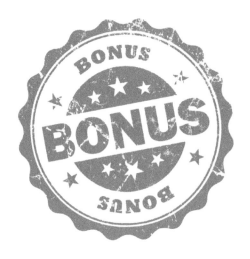

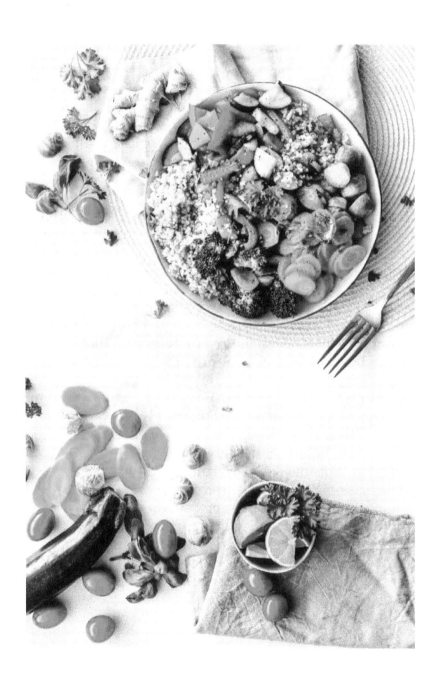

COPYRIGHT

Table of Contents

—

6

INTRODUCTION

When thinking about a diet or change in lifestyle, it's critical to think about the advantages and entanglements. If the diet won't profit you – what's the point? Yet additionally, if the symptoms are unmanageable, you might need to reconsider. Keto diets are more well-known than any time in recent memory with a high number of competitors changing to along these lines of eating/living. The Keto diet/method for living comprises of eating nourishments that are high in fat, moderate in protein and low in carbs. When on a Keto diet, the body adjusts from utilizing carbs to utilizing fats to consume vitality.

Here we take a gander at the advantages of the Keto diet, and for what reason is may be for you. Remember to find out about the reactions as well – we couldn't not have a reasonable contention, might we be able to!

1 – Improved body organization

Obviously, one of the principle reasons that individuals move to any diet is to improve their body shape and piece. The Keto diet has been demonstrated to diminish muscle versus fat and build fit weight, basically making somebody look more slender. When combined with quality preparing and lifting, the body organization can improve most prominently.

2 – Increased vitality levels

When you eat heaps of carbs for the duration of the day, your glucose levels go here and there. On the Keto diet, your vitality levels are bound to be reliable for the duration of the day as you're not getting the spikes in glucose. The perpetual stock of vitality from the high fats are probably going to keep you feeling stimulated and will stop those spikes. It is critical to call attention to however that when beginning on a Keto diet, your vitality levels might be lower because of weariness from the stun to your collection of eating less carbs.

—

3 – Can decrease awful skin

Eating a Keto diet has been demonstrated to help diminish skin inflammation and awful skin. As the Keto diet removes carbs and prepared nourishments which can have effect on gut health, many notice an improvement to their skin on this diet.

4 – Reduces cholesterol

Studies have discovered that the Keto diet can help decrease cholesterol and can make your heart healthier. Great cholesterol levels have been seen as expanded on the Keto diet, with terrible cholesterol being decreased.

5 – Reduces pulse

Low carb diets like the Keto Diet have been demonstrated to decrease pulse. Studies have demonstrated that eating less carbs can significantly affect decreasing this.

6 – Reduced fat particles in the body

Fat particles, otherwise called triglycerides will in general decrease drastically when on the Keto Diet. Expanded fat particles are often determined via starch utilization and fructose (sugar). When individuals cut carbs, their fat atoms significantly decrease. In actuality, when individuals cut fats in their diet, fat particles can really increment. This isn't an issue on the Keto diet which is high in fats.

7 – Reduced possibility of coronary illness

Instinctive fat will be fat under the skin in the stomach pit which lodges itself around the organs and can be hurtful. Low carb diets help to decrease instinctive fat, particularly that around the stomach pit. In the long haul, having less fat around there can lessen the danger of coronary illness and furthermore type 2 diabetes.

There are numerous advantages of going to a Keto Diet, yet recollect that this sort of diet ought to be considered as a long haul lifestyle change and not a prevailing fashion diet. The Keto diet is commended by numerous individuals for its outcomes in fat decrease and can likewise help with numerous other health upgrades.

KETO DIET RECIPES

You should seriously mull over diet a no-no on a ketogenic diet — yet reconsider. These keto diet recipes catch the equivalent springy, chewy, and toasty surface as common portions, all while keeping you all the more full and centered.

The most effective method to make the best keto diet

When getting ready keto diet recipes, pay special mind to low-carb ingredients that could add to brain haze and aggravation. Skip recipes that require regular dairy or yeast, and abstain from eating basic keto diet ingredients like psyllium husk, thickener, and nuts or nut margarines time after time — these can contain shape or disturb your gut. Grass-encouraged margarine, ghee, and coconut flour are the couple of exemptions that will at present produce an excellent portion.

From great cut diet to tortillas and sweet portions, keep these keto diet recipes close by for all your hardest carb desires:

Essential Keto Diet Recipes

This elastic, supplement stuffed portion utilizes heat-safe collagen peptides to give each chomp an additional protein support. With extra ingredients like almond flour and eggs, this formula makes a durable cut that holds up to sandwiches and spreads. In contrast to most recipes, this keto diet is an extraordinary 0 net carbs!

This collagen keto diet has zero net carbs per cut. It's sans dairy, sans grain, sans gluten, and the best part is that it utilizes heat-stable, grass-bolstered collagen protein as its essential element for giving the diet its structure. This keto diet is feathery, tasty, not excessively eggy, and this with zero net carbs per cut.

This keto diet formula is so natural to work with that the conceivable outcomes are inestimable. Use cuts simply like standard diet. It makes tasty virus sandwiches, French toast, garlic diet, and plunging diet. You can utilize it as a cheeseburger bun, make avocado toast bested with a poached egg, or truly anything you would do with customary diet.

What Makes This Keto Diet So Healthy?

If you've at any point taken a stab at preparing diet utilizing collagen protein as your primary "flour" source, then you realize that it is so testing to get it to remain cushioned and diet-like. My objective with this formula was to make a collagen-based keto diet that was as near standard diet as could reasonably be expected, with very low carbs and no dairy. This keto diet formula feels like I'm eating normal diet again and that can be useful, particularly when you're changing to a keto or Bulletproof diet.

Surprisingly better, this portion is standard size (not scaled down) and makes 12 liberal cuts. The macros per cut are around 77 calories, 5 grams of fat, 7 grams of protein, and 0 grams of net carbs (1 gram of carbs short 1 gram of fiber). You can without much of a stretch up the fat substance when expending this diet basically by slathering with grass-sustained ghee or margarine.

Add this keto diet formula to your armory of other great diet recipes that are paleo, keto and additionally Bulletproof. I think you'll think that its a great expansion to your formula box, and without a doubt when you're going ultra-low carb, this formula should ascend to the highest priority on your rundown.

———

COLLAGEN KETO DIET

Keto Collagen Diet Recipe Start to Finish: 1 hour and 50 minutes (10 minutes dynamic)
INGREDIENTS:
1/2 cup Unflavored Grass-Fed Collagen Protein
6 tablespoons almond flour (see formula notes beneath for sans nut substitute)
5 fed eggs, isolated
1 tablespoon unflavored fluid coconut oil
1 teaspoon without aluminum preparing powder
1 teaspoon thickener (see formula notes for substitute)
Squeeze Himalayan pink salt
Discretionary: squeeze of stevia

ALMOND FLOUR KETO DIET

With low-carb wash room staples like almond flour and Himalayan salt, this keto diet formula delivers an essential portion with no eggy taste at all. Isolating the eggs assists this with dieting stay feathery with no yeast — furthermore, each cut is just 1.25 net carbs. To remain increasingly Bulletproof, just use grass-nourished spread.

If you've been searching for what is completely the best keto diet formula on the web, then you've gone to the correct spot. How would I know it's the best? All things considered, I've attempted pretty much every keto diet formula in the course of recent years and chose that nothing posed a flavor like standard diet. A couple are great, however I needed flawlessness!

The best part about this formula is that it's basic, and once you have it down, you can reproduce this keto neighborly diet whenever you need. I've been making a low carb portion each Sunday for as long as not many weeks and would prescribe that to anybody. It's so pleasant to have a portion of diet available to you when you're on a low carb diet. It nearly wants to swindle. Look at this formula and start making the best keto diet you've at any point attempted today!

A Healthy Low Carb Diet Recipe

The mystery step in this formula that takes this without carb diet from great to extraordinary is the detachment of the eggs. You're going to need to isolate the yolks and the whites. The explanation behind this is we're going to whip the egg whites until they are soft. We're searching for delicate pinnacles. This will add some volume to the generally thick keto diet.

Beating the egg whites is the response to the thickness that accompanies making an almond flour diet. I've made endless prepared merchandise utilizing almond flour and the principle issue I've experienced is the manner by which thick the completed item is. The feathery egg whites as one with the high measurement of preparing powder work superbly of getting this portion decent and soft and including some air pockets into the portion. This makes for a superior tasting diet.

A few people approve of the well-known keto cloud diet recipes out there, however we needed something increasingly thick and filling. By adding the almond flour to the soft egg blend, you include progressively fat, protein, and calories making for a satisfying supper. Additionally, the surface and flavor is

What makes this the best keto diet formula is the way that you can utilize it a similar way you utilize normal diet. Sounds insane right? If you look for keto diet on Pinterest, or the web you'll locate a different formula for all that you should make.

In what capacity will you eat diet once more?

French toast – Try our Keto French Toast Recipe

Sandwiches

Diet garnishes

Avocado toast

BREAKFAST SANDWICH

You can do everything with this keto diet formula. You can even get insane and toss this diet in a nourishment processor and use it as Italian diet scraps. The conceivable outcomes are huge.

Your Low Carb Diet Replacement Has Arrived

The best part about this diet is that it makes it such a great amount of simpler to eat a low carb diet. Indeed, there are some savage monsters (kidding) that don't miss diet at all and are glad to simply eat bacon seven times each day, however if you're in any way similar to me, diet was a staple of your diet growing up despite everything you examine longing in your eyes when they drop that diet container in the table at family supper. I sympathize with your torment. This low carb diet formula is your comfort in times of dire need.

How would I dispose of the eggy taste?

There is a mellow eggy taste to this diet, which we happen to adore, however a few people don't care for it. We've tried two or three different approaches to dispense with it and here is the thing that we've thought of:

Stevia – It may sound insane, yet including a couple of drops of stevia to this formula is the most ideal approach to dispense with the eggy taste. Only a couple of drops will do! We regularly utilize 6 drops of stevia. That sum won't make the diet sweet to the taste by any stretch of the imagination, yet it will extraordinarily decrease the eggy taste.

Yeast – Adding a tablespoon of Active Dry Yeast to this formula can bring about a progressively conventional diet season. The yeast won't make the diet rise or anything since we're not utilizing sugar or gluten, yet the flavor will in any case come through.

Margarine – This may be the most ideal way ☺ Just add some tasty spread to the highest point of a cut and you will believe you're eating customary diet!

Is the keto diet without dairy?

———

This formula calls for dissolved margarine, however you can swap that out for whatever sort of without dairy fat you like best. Ghee, coconut oil, or avocado oil would all be extraordinary alternatives. Fill us in as to whether you attempt the swap and how your diet turns out.

Is the formula sans gluten?

Truly! This keto diet formula and the entirety of our other keto recipes are without gluten. The diet is made with finely ground almond flour rather than wheat flour, which implies you and your sans gluten companions can appreciate a cut

How would I store Keto Diet?

Cutting to arrange will be your most logical option from a timeframe of realistic usability stance. We pop the whole portion in the ice chest, either in a Tupperware compartment or a Ziploc sack and cut off cuts as we eat it. It will toward the end in the ice chest for 7-10 days.

How would I persuade my portion to be taller and fluffier?

The two significant issues that will prompt a level portion isn't whipping the egg whites and delicately collapsing them in OR utilizing almond supper rather than a finely ground almond flour. If you've had a go at everything and they don't appear to work for you, the following best alternative will be to make a bigger formula. Take a stab at making 1.5x this formula (it's anything but difficult to do utilizing the servings slide bar) and you'll have an a lot bigger portion.

Where to purchase Keto Diet close to me?

If you're not a devotee of preparing but rather you're a fanatic of eating diet, there are spots to get keto well-disposed diet nowadays. If you're fortunate, you might have the option to discover a portion of "Paleo Diet" in the cooler area at Whole Foods Market. This diet is going to cost you over $10 per portion, however it is made of good ingredients and is a couple of grams of carbs per cut. There's additionally gossipy tidbits about ALDI conveying another Zero-Carb diet, however it sells out quick and we haven't had the option to survey it. Ideally sooner rather than later there will be progressively nearby purchasing alternatives for low carb diet, yet until further notice, those are your lone choices.

Ingredients:

1/2 Cup Almond Flour

6 Large eggs Separated

1/4 cup Butter dissolved

3 tsp Baking powder

1/4 tsp Cream of Tartar It's alright if you don't have this

1 squeeze Pink Himalayan Salt

6 drops Liquid Stevia discretionary

Instructions:

Preheat stove to 375.

Separate the egg whites from the yolks. Add Cream of Tartar to the whites and beat until delicate pinnacles are accomplished.

In a nourishment processor join the egg yolks, 1/3 of the beaten egg whites, liquefied spread, almond flour, preparing powder and salt (Adding ~6 drops of fluid stevia to the player can help lessen the mellow egg taste). Blend until consolidated. This will be a knotty thick batter until the whites are included.

Include the staying 2/3 of the egg whites and delicately process until completely joined. Be mindful so as not to overmix as this is the thing that gives the diet it's volume!

Empty blend into a buttered 8x4 portion skillet. Heat for 30 minutes. Check with a toothpick to guarantee the diet is cooked through. Appreciate! 1 portion makes 20 cuts.

LOW-CARB KETO DIET

If you are delicate to lactose, attempt this keto diet formula. Rather than spread, the ingredients list calls for grass-encouraged ghee, which contains a lot of almost no lactose. With just four different ingredients, you can have this portion prepared to appreciate in well under 60 minutes. Besides, each tasty cut counts up to 3 net carbs.

Following a low carb diet doesn't need to mean lettuce-wrapped sandwiches forever! With this snappy diet formula, you can have French toast or barbecued cheddar sandwiches without sacrificing your carb tally.

The key to making a light and vaporous keto diet that can hold up to the toaster is utilizing a lot of eggs and healthy fat. Ghee is a butterfat that is cooked longer to sift through the milk solids, which makes it a lot simpler on the stomach related framework for individuals with lactose sensitivities. Grass-encouraged ghee is likewise high in the unsaturated fat CLA, which is useful for securing cells and diminishing oxidative harm.

If you need to make this diet taste increasingly like a wipe cake style diet to top with berries or Paleo dessert, include a teaspoon of stevia or other Paleo endorsed sugar to the player. To get a better surface, use almond flour rather than almond feast.

Start by beating the eggs utilizing a hand blender on fast. This joins air into the eggs, which makes an airier completed item. Next, beat in the liquefied ghee pursued by the dry ingredients to frame a hitter. Empty the blend into a portion container fixed with material paper and heat at 350°F for 40-45 minutes. Utilize a sharp knife to delicately expel the diet from container and utilizing the material paper to lift the diet out of the skillet. Cool for 10 minutes before cutting.

Tip: This diet additionally pairs as delectable flavorful or sweet biscuits. Mix in blueberries to make blueberry biscuits (remember, in any case, that the carb check will go up) or cleaved jalapeños and wholesome yeast for a fiery biscuit with a mushy bend.

Low Carb Keto Diet Recipe

Cut up this Paleo keto diet and heap it high with your preferred sandwich fixings.

Apparatuses

Portion dish

Material paper

Huge blending bowl

Hand blender

Spatula

Ingredients

7 huge eggs

1/2 cup dissolved ghee

2 cups almond flour

1 t preparing powder

1/4 t ocean salt

Instructions

Preheat the stove to 350°F and line a portion container with material paper covering the sides.

In a huge blending bowl, beat the eggs utilizing a hand blender on rapid for 1 moment. Include the dissolved ghee and beat until simply fused.

Decrease the speed to low and bit by bit include the rest of the ingredients until totally blended and the hitter is thick.

Empty the player into the readied skillet and spread with a spatula. Heat for 40-45 minutes, or until light brilliant dark colored on top.

Cool the diet on a cooling rack for 10 minutes before cutting.

PALEO COCONUT DIET

This paleo keto diet formula makes a tasty alternative for coconut darlings. For a low-object portion, mix coconut flour with ingredients like eggs, coconut oil, and salt — then heat away for a strong diet with just 1.3 net carbs per serving. Make this formula absolutely without nut (and increasingly Bulletproof) by swapping almond milk with full-fat canned coconut milk.

Everybody who realizes me is very much aware that when it comes to heating, there's nothing that I love more than decent, speedy, and simple recipes. Try not to misunderstand me - there's very a period and a spot for progressively expound extravagant preparing recipes. In any case, when I'm desiring something scrumptious crisp out of the broiler, more often than not I need something that I can prepare very fast that will taste delectable. That is actually why I love this formula for paleo coconut diet. It checks all the privilege boxes - brisk and simple to get ready, healthy every single common fixing, and staggeringly scrumptious.

I love everything about coconut — the particularly sweet flavor, how it's so effectively accessible in basically any store, and obviously, the wealth of healthy medium-chain triglyceride (MCT) fats contained inside them. (1) This coconut diet became animated when I needed to go through my remaining coconut flour from the last time I made lemon curd coconut hotcakes so I thought, why not make diet out of it utilizing one of my current recipes. Not surprisingly, no refined wheat flour was utilized, however you could never figure with how staggering this present diet's surface turns out subsequent to preparing.

Subsequent to combining your coconut flour with the salt and heating pop, turn your consideration towards setting up a wet blend for your diet batter. Join your six eggs, almond milk, and obviously, your softened coconut oil. Clearly, the coconut oil will add considerably more coconut goodness to your diet, however the unsweetened almond milk fits in this formula pleasantly too. It guarantees that this diet is sans dairy over being sans gluten, and it includes a pleasant measure of nutrients and minerals in with the general mish-mash also. In the wake of joining your wet blend, gradually include it into the coconut flour blend and you'll be good to go to start preparing.

Heating with Coconut Flour

Coconut flour can be dubious to work with from the outset. It absorbs a ton of dampness, so ensure you add a great deal of fluid to your player. If it's as thick as hotcake hitter, then it's excessively thick and will presumably wind up like a hockey puck in the wake of heating. The player should be too runny when utilizing coconut flour to guarantee it winds up sodden and cushioned.

There are hardly any things in life that will make your kitchen smell superior to the aroma of diet heating in the stove. On that note, there are not a lot of diets out there that I can appreciate eating plain. Typically I need to include either some kind of nut margarine or grass bolstered spread in any event. I'm glad to report that is not the situation with this formula — this coconut diet packs a terrific measure of scrumptious coconut season into every single chomp.

Ingredients

1/2 cup coconut flour

1/4 tsp salt

1/4 tsp preparing pop

6 eggs

¼ cup coconut oil, dissolved

¼ unsweetened almond milk

Bearings

———

Preheat stove to 350°F.

Line a 8×4 inch portion dish with material paper.

In a bowl consolidate the coconut flour, heating pop and salt.

In another bowl consolidate the eggs, drain and oil.

Gradually include the wet ingredients into the dry ingredients and blend until consolidated.

Empty the blend into the readied portion dish.

Heat for 40-50 minutes, or until a toothpick, embedded in the center confesses all.

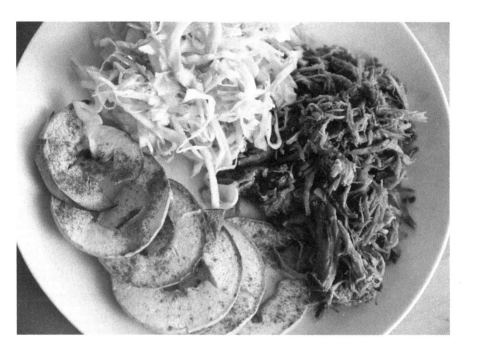

MACADAMIA NUT DIET

This keto diet formula makes an ideal external outside layer and delicate morsel, on account of high-fat macadamia nuts ground directly into the hitter. Mix nuts with eggs, coconut flour, heating pop, and apple juice vinegar, then prepare. That is it! Per cut, each serving runs 1 net carb — simply ensure you abstain from eating macadamias time after time to remain Bulletproof.

This macadamia nut diet is rich, cushioned and flexible. Tastes simply like conventional diet, and has a hard external layer and delicate inside! Ideal for those following a without gluten, sans grain, ketogenic, low-carb, Paleo or sans dairy lifestyle.

I've made a few diet recipes previously, however none very as delectable and near a conventional burden as this macadamia nut diet. This formula certainly takes the cake (diet), when it comes to low-carb and without gluten diets.

This formula was motivated by the woman in the narrative "The Magic Pill" who made a heap of diet utilizing ground macadamia nuts. I didn't have the foggiest idea about this was a THING. When I perceived how mind blowing her diet turned out, I realized I needed to attempt it.

So I utilized the macadamia nut thought and chose to explore a piece until I found the one I enjoyed best. I accept the formula in the narrative utilized a lot of coconut spread. While I do like me some coconut margarine, I attempted to keep this formula somewhat progressively moderate. That stuff is upwards of $10 a container, and you need bountiful sums for a portion of diet!

So as I referenced over, the base of this formula is ground macadamia nuts. I utilized 5 oz, which for my situation is an entire pack. Essentially crush them in a nourishment processor or blender until they structure a nut margarine.

If you're utilizing a blender, you may need to add some fluid to get it to mix completely.

You can begin including the eggs each in turn until there is sufficient fluid to mix everything up. Include the remainder of the eggs and mix until well-consolidated. Blend in the coconut flour, heating pop and apple juice vinegar.

Shower a diet container and include the batter. Prepare in the broiler for 30-40 minutes or until the outside is decent and firm. Permit to cool to room temperature.

INGREDIENTS

5 oz macadamia nuts I utilized the Royal Hawaiian brand

5 enormous eggs

1/4 cup coconut flour (28 g)

1/2 teaspoon heating pop

1/2 teaspoon apple juice vinegar

This macadamia nut diet is rich, cushioned and adaptable. Tastes simply like conventional diet, and has a dried up external layer and delicate inside! Ideal for those following a sans gluten, sans grain, ketogenic, low-carb, Paleo or sans dairy lifestyle.

INSTRUCTIONS

Preheat broiler to 350F.

To a blender or nourishment processor, include macadamia nuts and heartbeat until it turns into a nut spread. If your blender doesn't work superbly without fluid, include eggs each in turn until the consistency is that of a nut spread.

Scratch drawbacks of blender or nourishment processor, and include remaining eggs. Mix until well-consolidated.

Include coconut flour, preparing pop and apple juice vinegar and heartbeat until fused.

Oil a standard-size diet container and include player. Smooth surface of player and spot on base rack of broiler for 30-40 minutes, or until the top is brilliant darker.

Expel from broiler and permit to cool in prospect 20 minutes before expelling.

Will store in a hermetically sealed compartment at room temperature for 3-4 days at room temperature, or for multi week in the cooler.

LOW-CARB GARLIC and HERB FOCACCIA

A mix of heating pop, lemon squeeze, and preparing powder dispenses with the requirement for yeast in this bubbly keto diet formula. With huge amounts of Italian seasonings, olive oil, and flaky salt sprinkled on top, you'll need to incorporate this portion with each supper. Each liberal cut is 3 net carbs — and to remain progressively Bulletproof, essentially abstain from eating garlic and thickener time and again.

Conventional focaccia is a yeast diet that is like pizza batter and is made for cutting up and presenting with your principle course. Despite the fact that I have utilized yeast in keto and low carb diet recipes, I didn't need the sit tight for a yeasty keto diet to confirmation and rise this time.

To supplant the yeast in the raising procedure, I utilized twofold activity preparing powder and heating soft drink + lemon juice. The piece in this specific formula is somewhat denser than customary focaccia and delicate yet brittle—and it's on purpose! The underlying groups were excessively thick and chewy, however not positively, and it detracted from the stunning kinds of garlic, salt, and basil. SO I skirted the psyllium husk fiber to accomplish a decent surface without the dull dark colored/purple shade that an excess of psyllium brings. For me, despite the fact that this is all out con artist's focaccia, it hits the spot and shields me from thumping over a diet store and going into a gluten-unconsciousness

Ingredients

DRY INGREDIENTS

1 cup Almond Flour

1/4 cup Coconut Flour

1/2 tsp Xanthan Gum

1 tsp Garlic Powder

1 tsp Flaky Salt

1/2 tsp Baking Soda

1/2 tsp Baking Powder

Falk Salt, discretionary to decorate

WET INGREDIENTS

2 eggs

1 tbsp Lemon Juice

2 tsp Olive oil + 2 tbsp Olive Oil to sprinkle

Instructions

Warmth broiler to 350 and line a heating plate or 8-inch round dish with material.

Whisk together the dry ingredients ensuring there are no irregularities.

Beat the egg, lemon squeeze, and oil until joined.

Blend the wet and the dry together, working rapidly, and scoop the batter into your skillet.

***Make sure not to blend the wet and dry until you are prepared to place the diet in the stove because the raising response starts once it is blended!!!

Smooth the top and edges with a spatula plunged in water (or your hands) then utilize your finger to dimple the mixture. Try not to be hesitant to dive deep on the dimples! Once more, a little water shields it from staying.

Prepare secured for around 10 minutes. Shower with Olive Oil heat for an extra 10-15 minutes revealing to darker tenderly.

Top with flaky salt, olive oil (discretionary), a scramble of Italian flavoring and new basil. Let cool totally before cutting for ideal surface!!

CAULIFLOWER DIET WITH GARLIC AND HERBS

Sneak a few veggies into your keto diet with this straightforward, delightful formula. A mix of riced cauliflower and coconut flour makes a persuading substitute for dull diet ingredients, while ocean salt and herbs include an exquisite touch. To remain Bulletproof on this 3-carb diet, use grass-encouraged margarine and abstain from eating garlic time and again.

One normal demand I hear a great deal in the low carb network is keto low carb diet recipes. Trust me, I get it! Some of the time you simply need some cut diet for a basic sandwich. Or on the other hand some low carb garlic diet. My typical go-to's are low carb diet with almond flour or keto low carb fathead bagels, yet I've been searching for something somewhat lighter. That is the place this cauliflower diet formula comes in.

Would you be able to accept that this cauliflower diet with garlic and herbs has just 108 calories and 3g net carbs per cut? That's right, it's valid. I don't check calories, yet I do get a kick out of the chance to have light choices accessible. This keto cloud diet is another extraordinary lighter decision for low carb diet.

Cauliflower tortillas and cauliflower diet sticks are really normal, so why not basic cauliflower diet, isn't that so? Cauliflower is such a valuable sub for starches in nourishments, I can't trust I didn't think about this sooner. It's an extraordinary method to make your low carb diet on the lighter side – as far as carbs, yet calories as well.

Despite the fact that the cuts aren't extremely enormous, they are still huge enough for a decent sandwich. You can duplicate the formula by 1.5, or even twofold it, if you favor bigger cuts. You can likewise cut the diet more slender, if wanted, to lessen the carbs more.

One of my preferred approaches to utilize cauliflower diet is for flame broiled cheddar. The flavors work so well together! The best part is, broiling it a little makes a heavenly hard outside.

That is only one thought. You truly can eat this diet in for the most part similar ways you'd eat some other portion of diet. Simply take a gander at those cuts. Am I the one in particular that needs to make an enormous BLT sandwich with them, similar to the present moment?

If it's not clear yet, my unique expectation for a cauliflower diet portion was a lighter, low carb sandwich diet. It functions admirably for that reason, however it's somewhat more dry and thick than some other low carb diet recipes. It tastes best with a spread, or sauces on your sandwich.

When I saw this, it jumped out at me a somewhat drier cauliflower diet makes an extraordinary possibility for low carb garlic diet! Furthermore, since a low carb garlic diet formula was on my rundown to make at any rate, I was glad to consolidate the two.

I quickly bested a few cuts with margarine, garlic, and parsley, alongside a sprinkle of ocean salt. Only 10 minutes in a hot broiler, and voila! Cauliflower diet transformed into low carb garlic diet! Who knew?!

INGREDIENTS

Snap underlined ingredients to get them!

3 cup Cauliflower ("riced" utilizing nourishment processor*)

10 enormous Egg (isolated)

1/4 tsp Cream of tartar (discretionary)

1/4 cup Coconut flour

1/2 tbsp sans gluten heating powder

1 tsp Sea salt

6 tbsp Butter (unsalted, estimated strong, then liquefied; can utilize ghee for sans dairy)

6 cloves Garlic (minced)

1 tbsp Fresh rosemary (cleaved)

1 tbsp Fresh parsley (cleaved)

INSTRUCTIONS

Formula TIPS + VIDEO in the post above, sustenance data + formula notes beneath!

Preheat the broiler to 350 degrees F (177 degrees C). Line a 9x5 in (23x13 cm) portion container with material paper.

Steam the riced cauliflower. You can do this in the microwave (cooked for 3-4 minutes, shrouded in plastic) OR in a steamer bin over water on the stove (line with cheesecloth if the openings in the steamer bushel are too huge, and steam for a couple of moments). The two different ways, steam until the cauliflower is delicate and delicate. Enable the cauliflower to cool enough to deal with.

Then, use a hand blender to beat the egg whites and cream of tartar until stiff tops structure.

Spot the coconut flour, preparing powder, ocean salt, egg yolks, liquefied margarine, garlic, and 1/4 of the whipped egg whites in a nourishment processor.

When the cauliflower has cooled enough to deal with, envelop it by kitchen towel and press a few times to discharge however much dampness as could reasonably be expected. (This is significant - the final product ought to be exceptionally dry and bunch together.) Add the cauliflower to the nourishment processor. Procedure until all around consolidated. (Blend will be thick and somewhat brittle.)

Add the rest of the egg whites to the nourishment processor. Crease in only a bit, to make it simpler to process. Heartbeat a couple of times until simply fused. (Blend will be feathery.) Fold in the slashed parsley and rosemary. (Don't overmix to abstain from separating the egg whites excessively.)

Move the player into the lined preparing skillet. Smooth the top and round somewhat. If wanted, you can squeeze more herbs into the top (discretionary).

Heat for around 45-50 minutes, until the top is brilliant. Cool totally before evacuating and cutting.

Instructions to Make Buttered Low Carb Garlic Diet (discretionary): Top cuts liberally with margarine, minced garlic, new parsley, and a little ocean salt. Prepare in a preheated broiler at 450 degrees F (233 degrees C) for around 10 minutes. If you need it progressively cooked, place under the grill for a few minutes.

COCONUT FLOUR FLATDIET

Utilize this keto diet for wraps, plunges, curries, and anyplace else you'd regularly utilize a naan-style diet. This formula makes delicious, malleable diet without any eggs and just 2.6 net carbs per serving. To keep it increasingly Bulletproof, swap olive oil with avocado oil or coconut oil, and abstain from eating psyllium husk time after time.

Coconut flour flatdiet otherwise called coconut flour tortillas are simple, delicate and adaptable keto tortilla with just 2.6 g net carbs per serve.

A standout amongst other vegetarian keto diet recipes ideal for lunch sandwich wraps or to fill in as a side dish to your curry. Reward, those coconut flour keto diet have no eggs, no dairy or cheddar and can be incorporated on a veggie lover keto diet.

IS COCONUT FLOUR GOOD FOR KETO DIET?

Truly, coconut flour is a standout amongst other low carb flour for keto heating including for keto diets or keto wraps with just 21 g net carbs per 100 g. Note that coconut flour is exceptionally permeable and keto recipes utilize just a little measure of it, a serve is typically second rate compared to 1/2 cup for every formula, adding just 10g net carb to the formula, as in those coconut flour tortillas.

WHAT NUMBER OF CARBS ARE IN COCONUT FLOUR?

Coconut flour contains 38 g of non-edible fiber per 100 g which implies there is just 21 g net carbs per 100 g. Remember that normal flour contains 74 g net carbs implying that coconut flour has 3.5 occasions less carbs than customary white flour.

COCONUT FLOUR TORTILLAS INGREDIENTS

As notice over, those Coconut flour tortillas are anything but difficult to make. All you need are hardly any straightforward keto veggie lover ingredients:

Coconut flour – obviously DONT utilize other flour, it is the base fixing to make coconut flour flatdiet. Coconut flour is low carb, high fiber flour and that is the way to make a tasty low carb diet. Psyllium husk – same here you MUST utilize psyllium husk. As the formula is eggless the husk is the thing that unites the flour, make a delicate and somewhat chewy diet as a customary flatdiet or roti. It is zero net carb nourishment as it is essentially 100% fiber.

Heating pop – I am not utilizing a lot however it is the thing that I thought carries the light cushy surface to the flatdiet, don't hesitate to discard the formula will even now work

Salt – discretionary however I love my diet marginally salty

Water – I utilized tepid water, think shower temperature. I utilized faucet water about 38C

Olive oil – some other vegetable oil can be used in this formula. Other healthy choice would be avocado oil, sunflower oil or softened coconut oil.

The mixture is quite simple to make. Essentially bring all the dry ingredients into a blending bowl and consolidate in with the wet ingredients, any request works! I thought that it was simpler to legitimately massage the batter by hands as it isn't clingy or chaotic. It unites the ingredients effectively. It is clammy from the outset yet it gets dryer following 1 moment. Then, rest the entire batter in the bowl for 10 minutes to give the psyllium a chance to husk suck the dampness and make a versatile delicate mixture.

GLUTEN FREE FLATDIET
Coconut flour flatdiet are by definition veggie lover gluten free flatdiet has they contains no wheat, no eggs, no margarine or cheddar. Coconut flour and psyllium husk make the most flavorful gluten free flatdiet surface that won't break when filled.

INSTRUCTIONS TO SHAPE ROUND COCONUT FLOUR TORTILLAS ?

Pursue the means underneath to shape beautiful round coconut flour tortillas. Something else, don't hesitate to shape the coconut flour diet has you like, square, square shape anything you extravagant will work!

Cut the batter ball into 4 even pieces.

Roll every piece in a ball, place this ball between two bit of material paper

Press the ball with your hand to crush it between the paper and start rolling.

Move as slender as you can imagine your diet – remember that they puff a piece when cooking so meager is alright ! mine are too slight and they don't break

Strip off the top bit of paper

Discretionary – use a top or any balance shape to cut beautiful round flatdiet and keep the outside batter to change more diet.

Flip over the flatdiet onto a hot nonstick skillet, strip off the last bit of paper cautiously to discharge the diet.

Cook 2-3 minutes on the two sides.

VEGETARIAN KETO DIET RECIPES TIPS AND TRICKS

Veggie lover keto diet recipes don't utilize eggs, cheddar or dairy. It doesn't mean the formula is confuse. This coconut flour diet batter is really simple to work with and I never had any issue with this formula. Anyway I recorded beneath the two different ways it could turn out badly, why and what to do to assist you with making the most flavorful coconut flatdiet right away! Note that the mixture must be delicate, flexible, not clingy to your hands. You should have the option to shape a bundle of mixture before saving for 10 moment. The mixture must be somewhat delicate, versatile and a piece dryer in the wake of resting time – which means not clingy !

Excessively damp, can't frame a ball ?

That is alright, include somewhat more psyllium husk include this progressively 1/2 teaspoon at once! Massage the batter and continue including more husk until it meets up into a mixture. Ensure you ply at any rate 1 moment between every expansion to ensure the husk adsorb the dampness and unite the batter. You shouldn't require more than 1 teaspoon extra ! Formula consistently functions admirably for me without including any additional husk.

Excessively brittle, excessively dry?

You likely added to a lot of coconut flour or yours wasn't fine – once in a while coconut flour frames little protuberances that make it difficult to unequivocally quantify in a cup. Basically include more water 1 teaspoon at once, work 30 sec and perceive how it goes. I additionally suggest estimating the coconut flour in the wake of expelling any irregularity in your bunch – if any. Essentially utilize a fork to crush them, then measure.

HOW TO HEAT FLATDIET?
Skillet tips

—

A nonstick tefal crepe dish or flapjack iron is the best to cook or warm your flatdiet. Somewhat oil your skillet with 1 teaspoon of olive oil, rub onto a bit of permeable paper. You need the dish to be oiled yet no oil drop ought to remind in the skillet or your fry the flatdiet.

WHAT GOES GOOD ON FLATDIET?
Any of your preferred sandwich wraps can be made with those keto coconut flour flatdiet. Anything that you are needing can be made with a flatdiet like:
BLT sandwich wraps – Bacon, lettuce, tomatoes
Chicken Souvlaki wraps
Fish wraps
Ham and cheddar wraps
Vegetarian TLT wraps – tempeh or tofu, lettuce, tomatoes
INGREDIENTS
2 tablespoons psyllium husk (9g)
1/2 cup coconut flour fine, crisp, no protuberances (60g)
1 cup tepid water (240ml)
1 tablespoon olive oil (15ml)
1/4 teaspoons heating pop
1/4 teaspoons salt - discretionary
COOKING
1 teaspoon olive oil to rub/oil the nonstick skillet
INSTRUCTIONS
MAKE THE DOUGH
In a medium blending bowl, join the psyllium husk and coconut flour (if knots are in your flour utilize a fork to crush them BEFORE estimating the flour, sum must be exact).
Include the tepid water (I utilized faucet water about 40C/shower temperature), olive oil, and heating pop. Give a decent mix with a spatula, then utilize your hands to work the batter. Include salt now if you need. I never include the salt in contact with heating soft drink to abstain from deactivating the leading operator.

Ply for 1 moment. The batter is clammy and it gets milder and somewhat dryer as you go. It should meet up effectively to frame a batter as on my image. If not, excessively clingy, include more husk, 1/2 teaspoon at once, manipulate for 30 sec and perceive how it goes. The batter will consistently be somewhat soggy yet it shouldn't adhere to your hands by any means. It must meet up as a batter.

Put aside 10 moment in the blending bowl.

Presently the mixture must be delicate, flexible and hold well together, it is good to go.

Move/SHAPE THE FLATDIET

Cut the mixture into 4 even pieces, fold every piece into a little ball.

Spot one of the mixture ball between two bits of material paper, press the ball with your hand palm to adhere it well to the paper and start moving with a moving pin as slim as you can imagine a diet. My diets are 20 cm distance across (8 inches) and I made 6 flatdiet with this formula.

Un strip the main layer of material paper from your flatdiet. Utilize a top to remove round flatdiet. Keep the outside mixture to change a ball and move more flatdiet - that is the way I make 2 additional flatdiet from the 4 balls above!

COOK IN NON STICK PAN

Warm a nonstick tefal crepe/flapjack container under medium/high warmth or use any nonstick skillet of your decision, the one you would use for your hotcakes. Include one teaspoon of olive oil or vegetable oil of your decision onto a bit of retentive paper. Rub the outside of the skillet to ensure it is somewhat oiled. Try not to leave any drops of oil or the diet will broil!

Flip over the flatdiet on the hot dish and strip off cautiously the last bit of material paper.

Cook for 2-3 minutes on the primary side, flip over utilizing a spatula and cook for 1-2 increasingly minute on the opposite side.

Chill off the flatdiet on a plate and use as a sandwich wrap later or appreciate hot as a side dish. I suggest a shower of olive oil, squashed garlic and herbs before serving ! (discretionary however delish!)

Rehash the moving, cooking for the following 3 flatdiet. Ensure you rub the oiled spongy paper onto the pot each opportunity to maintain a strategic distance from the diet to adhere to the container.

Store in the wash room in a water/air proof box or on a plate secured with cling wrap to keep them delicate, for as long as 3 days.

Rewarm in a similar dish or if you need to give them somewhat fresh rewarm in the hot stove on a heating sheet for 1-2 minutes at 150C.

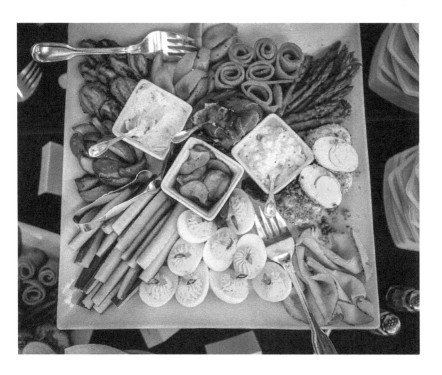

CAULIFLOWER TORTILLAS

This paleo, keto diet elective uses cauliflower as a base for adaptable, delightful tortillas. Crushing the dampness out of the riced cauliflower, in addition to including eggs, keeps these tortillas solid enough for taco fillings or wraps. To remain progressively Bulletproof, steam cauliflower as opposed to microwaving.

This formula may come as a stun to you, however today I'm demonstrating how to make tortillas out of cauliflower... indeed, these are Cauliflower Tortillas!

Watch the snappy, how-to video telling you the best way to make Cauliflower Tortillas, then print out the total formula toward the finish of this post so you can make them at home.

It starts with cauliflower that has been crushed into cous-cous-like granules in your nourishment processor. A few people have referenced in the remarks that they've had achievement utilizing as of now riced cauliflower as opposed to handling a head of cauliflower. When it's in this express, a short stretch in the microwave softens it up. If you don't claim a microwave, simply steam it on the stove.

When cauliflower is cooked, the dampness turns out in full power. Enveloped by cheesecloth or a meager dishtowel, you can tenderly press out the dampness. It's imperative to press out ALL of the dampness!

The disintegrated cauliflower is blended in with egg, salt and pepper (I include crisp cilantro and lime juice). If you are vegetarian, or if you are sensitive to eggs... perusers have referenced that they substitute flax eggs with no issue.

This blend is formed into "tortillas" and prepared first on one side and afterward on the other.

Then the Cauliflower Tortillas are set on a rack for a touch of cooling.

The last brisk advance in the formula is hurling them in a warming skillet for a touch of cooking and crisping on each side.

Heap of Cauliflower Tortillas

That is it! I appreciate these Cauliflower Tortillas straight out of the search for gold. I additionally appreciate them with a little cheddar softened on top like a quesadilla. They're additionally great in the first part of the day with a fried egg and eaten like a taco.

They are to some degree flexible to curve and load up with a limited quantity of filling for tacos, however they are definitely immaculate to eat independent from anyone else as well. I prescribe eating them "tostada-style" because they may tear when attempting to twist like a taco. Have a go at garnish them with this Best Ground Beef Taco Meat.

Heap of Cauliflower Tortillas

Would you be able to taste the cauliflower? I'd state, yes. If you've at any point tested the cauliflower pizza covering, you'll probably likewise be an enthusiast of Cauliflower Tortillas. You may likewise prefer to attempt my Zucchini Pizza Crust as well!

WOULD YOU BE ABLE TO FREEZE CAULIFLOWER TORTILLAS?

This is a regularly posed inquiry, yet I haven't had a go at solidifying them so I don't know how well that functions. My supposition is that they would be fine. Simply heat them in a hot skillet to warm them up and make them flexible once more.

Attempt them, and let me comprehend what you think.

INGREDIENTS

3/4 huge head cauliflower (or two cups riced)

2 huge eggs (Vegans, sub flax eggs)

1/4 cup hacked crisp cilantro

1/2 medium lime, squeezed and zested

salt and pepper, to taste

INSTRUCTIONS

Preheat the stove to 375 degrees F., and line a heating sheet with material paper.

Trim the cauliflower, cut it into little, uniform pieces, and heartbeat in a nourishment processor in clumps until you get a couscous-like consistency. The finely riced cauliflower should make around 2 cups stuffed.

Spot the cauliflower in a microwave-safe bowl and microwave for 2 minutes, then mix and microwave again for an additional 2 minutes. If you don't utilize a microwave, a steamer works similarly also. Spot the cauliflower in a fine cheesecloth or dainty dishtowel and crush out however much fluid as could reasonably be expected, being mindful so as not to consume yourself. Dishwashing gloves are recommended as it is hot.

In a medium bowl, whisk the eggs. Include cauliflower, cilantro, lime, salt and pepper. Blend until very much consolidated. Utilize your hands to shape 6 little "tortillas" on the material paper.

Prepare for 10 minutes, cautiously flip every tortilla, and come back to the stove for an extra 5 to 7 minutes, or until totally set. Spot tortillas on a wire rack to cool somewhat.

Warmth a medium-sized skillet on medium. Spot a heated tortilla in the dish, pushing down somewhat, and darker for 1 to 2 minutes on each side. Rehash with outstanding tortillas.

RICH AND SOFT SKILLET FLATDIET

No stove, no issue: You can in any case make keto diet directly from your skillet with this formula. Since it utilizes basic ingredients and cooks in bunches from your stovetop, you won't need to stand by long for diet to cool before eating up it.

Ingredients

1 cup Almond Flour

2 tbsp Coconut Flour

2 tsp Xanthan Gum

1/2 tsp Baking Powder

1/2 tsp Falk Salt

1 Whole Egg + 1 Egg White

1 tbsp Water

1 tbsp Oil for singing

1 tbsp softened Butter-for slathering

Instructions

Whisk together the dry ingredients (flours, thickener, preparing powder, salt) until very much consolidated.

Include the egg and egg white and beat tenderly into the flour to join. The batter will start to shape.

Include the tablespoon of water and start to work the batter to permit the flour and thickener to assimilate the dampness.

Cut the mixture in 4 equivalent parts and press each area out with stick wrap. Watch the video for instructions!

Warmth an enormous skillet over medium warmth and include oil.

Fry every flatdiet for around 1 min on each side.

Brush with spread (while hot) and embellish with salt and slashed parsley.

TURMERIC CAULIFLOWER BUNS

Cauliflower makes a scrumptious substitution in low-carb recipes, and this keto diet is no special case. Riced cauliflower mixes with coconut flour and mitigating turmeric to make hot and soft buns with no veggie taste. To remain increasingly Bulletproof, steam cauliflower as opposed to microwaving and avoid the dark pepper.

These 4-Ingredient Turmeric Cauliflower Buns are a simple sans grain, low-carb, and too healthy side dish.

INGREDIENTS

1 medium head of cauliflower or around 2 cups of immovably pressed cauliflower rice (see bearings for making the cauliflower rice)

2 eggs

2 tablespoons coconut flour

¼ teaspoon ground turmeric

squeeze every one of salt and pepper

INSTRUCTIONS

Preheat broiler to 400°F.

Line a heating sheet with material paper and put in a safe spot.

Take your cauliflower and utilize a sharp knife to remove the base. Draw off any green parts and utilize your hands to break the cauliflower into florets. Give the florets a speedy wash and pat dry.

Next, make cauliflower rice by setting the florets into the bowl of a nourishment processor with the "S" sharp edge. Heartbeat for around 30 seconds until the cauliflower is about the size of rice. You ought to have around two cups of solidly pressed cauliflower rice.

Spot the cauliflower rice into a microwavable-safe bowl with about a teaspoon of water. Spread with saran wrap and jab a couple of gaps to allow the to steam escape. Microwave the cauliflower rice for around 3 minutes. Then again, you can steam the cauliflower rice on the stovetop in a steamer container.

Reveal the bowl and let the cauliflower rice cool for around 5 minutes. Then, utilize a huge spoon to put the cauliflower rice into a nut milk pack or a perfect kitchen towel. Press the overabundance dampness out, being mindful so as not to consume your hands.

Empty the cauliflower rice into a medium blending bowl and mix in the eggs, turmeric, and a touch of salt and dark pepper.

Utilize your hands to frame the blend into 6 buns, setting them on the preparing sheet.

Heat for 25-30 minutes or until the top turns out to be somewhat carmelized.

The cauliflower buns are best taught hot a thing or two out of the stove. They don't refrigerate or re-heat well (they will get soft), however they are scrumptious to the point that you'll no uncertainty destroy them right!

LOW-CARB ALMOND FLOUR BISCUITS

With five ingredients and 10 minutes of prep, this keto diet demonstrates that anybody can make keto diet. This formula makes rich moves with almond flour as the principle fixing, and every one runs just 2 net carbs. Keep this formula increasingly Bulletproof with grass-sustained spread or ghee.

Who else does feast prep on Sundays? I can't be the one and only one! Furthermore, low carb almond flour diet rolls show up in my prep.

A greater amount of you are taking a gander at recipes here at Wholesome Yum on Sunday than some other day of the week. Unmistakably, huge numbers of you were insane occupied in the kitchen yesterday.

I need to state I thoroughly concur with you – Sunday is the greatest day to cook for the week ahead. Since these paleo scones with almond flour have been in my week after week turn for as long as month, I couldn't stand by any more drawn out to share them!

Sunday supper prep has gotten an encouraging daily schedule for me.

My family doesn't as a rule have solid plans toward the beginning of the day that day, so I inquire as to whether she needs to cook with me. She screeches in charm inevitably! She adores sitting on the kitchen counter as I do my cooking. I let her transform over estimating cups into a bowl or mix utilizing a major spoon. Cooking is so sweet with your children!

As buzzword as it sounds, it feels like she's growing up excessively quick. The time we spend together in the kitchen is simply inestimable. It feels like minutes solidified in time.

Also, weekdays get so occupied for a considerable lot of us. Having a few parts of suppers all set ahead of time is a gigantic help and makes for simple weeknight dinners that are as yet healthy.

—

44

After I made these almond flour diet rolls just because, I wished I'd done it sooner. Not exclusively were they scrumptiously rich and fulfilling, yet having them close by all week was so helpful! I carried them to work, served them with supper, and even consolidated them into snacks. What might you use them during the current week?

Treat Scoop – Using a treat scoop is a simple method to frame your rolls.

Huge Baking Sheet – This heating sheet will work extraordinary for making these tasty keto rolls.

INGREDIENTS

2 cup Blanched almond flour

2 tsp sans gluten heating powder

1/2 tsp Sea salt

2 enormous Egg (beaten)

1/3 cup Butter (estimated strong, then liquefied; can utilize ghee or coconut oil for sans dairy)

INSTRUCTIONS

Formula TIPS + VIDEO in the post above, sustenance data + formula notes underneath!

Preheat the broiler to 350 degrees F (177 degrees C). Line a heating sheet with material paper.

Combine dry ingredients in an enormous bowl. Mix in wet ingredients.

Scoop tablespoonful of the mixture onto the lined heating sheet (a treat scoop is the quickest way). Structure into adjusted roll shapes (level somewhat with your fingers).

Heat for around 15 minutes, until firm and brilliant. Cool on the heating sheet.

CRANBERRY JALAPEÑO "CORNDIET" MUFFINS

This keto diet formula conveys sweet warmth with no corn at all — rather, it utilizes a mix of coconut flour and sugar to catch a similar taste and surface for around 3 net carbs per serving. Include new cranberries and jalapeño cuts for a fun turn that sets well with occasion suppers. To keep this formula increasingly Bulletproof, use grass-nourished spread, swap almond milk with full-fat canned coconut milk, and skirt the peppers if you have a nightshade affectability.

Cranberries are such an occasional thing and, if you consider it a piece, you need to ask why. In this period of present day innovation and transportation, every single other berry are accessible all year. Full strawberries and ready raspberries are staying there on the produce stands even in the dead of winter, yet crisp cranberries show up in October and are for the most part off the racks by Christmas. I don't have the foggiest idea whether it's just because of buyer request and that individuals just think to purchase cranberries in the fall, or if they don't develop well in the hotter climes of Florida or California and in this manner really are just occasionally accessible. I realize that they require an unforgiving and acidic boggy condition, one that we happen to have a lot of in New England, and that might be the reason for their limited geology and time allotment. Whatever the explanation, I like my cranberries all year and I normally stock up and keep a few sacks in my cooler for spring and late spring cranberry longings

---

In any case, regardless I get energized when cranberry season moves around, because with it comes all that I love about fall. The cooler temperatures and the radiant foliage simply go inseparably with a hankering for everything cranberry. This year, I was truly the principal individual to purchase a pack of crisp cranberries at my nearby market. I had this specific formula at the top of the priority list when I showed up, yet I was concerned that I was too soon and that they wouldn't have any in stock yet. I had fingers crossed that they were in any event conveying some solidified cranberries in the cooler path. Be that as it may, similarly as I strolled into the produce area, I saw a staff part dealing with a regular showcase of cranberries with a few cartons of the ruby red natural product. He had scarcely figured out how to heap up a couple of them before I strolled over and got a sack. Obviously my occasional cranberry yearnings were consummately planned.

A year ago I'd made some vanilla bean cupcakes with coconut flour for my little girl's birthday. I made a tremendous bunch with the goal of utilizing them for the other children's birthday events also, yet at last, we ate a significant number of them unfrosted as breakfast biscuits. What's more, all things considered, they helped me a lot to remember corndiet. The surface was somewhat less grainy because of the finely ground coconut flour yet the flavor was fundamentally the same as an improved corndiet formula. That idea latched onto my subconscious mind, I surmise, so when I had a hankering for an increasingly appetizing, corndiet-like biscuit, I realized those cupcakes would be anything but difficult to adjust. I diminished the sugar and the vanilla, and I included some hacked cranberries and jalapeño for a fun little bend. They were tasty and would be an ideal expansion to any Thanksgiving table.

Low carb, sans grain biscuits that pose a flavor like corndiet! Made with coconut flour and overflowing with cranberries and jalapeño, these scrumptious biscuits would make an extraordinary expansion to any Thanksgiving table.

Course: Side Dish
Food: Diet
Servings: 12 biscuits
Calories: 157 kcal
Ingredients
1 cup coconut flour (I utilized Bob's Red Mill)
1/3 cup Swerve Sweetener or other erythritol
1 tbsp heating powder
1/2 tsp salt
7 enormous eggs, delicately beaten
1 cup unsweetened almond milk
1/2 cup margarine, dissolved OR avocado oil
1/2 tsp vanilla
1 cup crisp cranberries, cut down the middle
3 tbsp minced jalapeño peppers
1 jalapeño, seeds evacuated, cut into 12 cuts, for embellish
Instructions
Preheat broiler to 325F and oil a biscuit tin well or fix with paper liners.

In a medium bowl, whisk together coconut flour, sugar, heating powder and salt. Separate any bunches with the back of a fork.

Mix in eggs, dissolved spread and almond drain and mix enthusiastically. Mix in vanilla concentrate and keep on mixing until blend is smooth and very much consolidated. Mix in cleaved cranberries and jalapeños.

Gap player equally among arranged biscuit cups and spot one cut of jalapeño over each.

Heat 25 to 30 minutes or until tops are set and an analyzer embedded in the inside confesses all. Let cool 10 minutes in skillet, then move to a wire rack to cool totally.

KETO BAGELS

Not at all like other low-carb bagels that require traditional cheddar to tie them together, this keto diet formula utilizes psyllium husk to make the equivalent thick surface. You might need to appreciate these bagels split down the middle, since every one contains 7 net carbs. Keep each chomp increasingly Bulletproof and use grass-encouraged ghee, swap white vinegar for apple juice vinegar, exchange olive oil for avocado oil, and abstain from eating psyllium, garlic, or sesame seeds time and again.

If you've at any point been around somebody preparing for a long distance race, you've most likely seen them beating carbs. Heaps of carbs.

What's more, if you're similar to me, you most likely need to tear the bagels directly out of their hands and appreciate them yourself.

I have a superior thought. Disregard your sprinter companions and get your fix with this Keto bagel formula.

Removing the Carbs From Bagels

When I consider carbs, I consider bagels. That is to say, they don't give out plate of mixed greens toward the finish of a race.

So how on the planet do you make a bagel Keto? Is it actually a bagel if it doesn't have every one of those carbs?

Indeed, and it's far and away superior.

You recover a bagel in your ownership, and your body doesn't get the stun of somewhere in the range of 48 grams of carbs.

I had to roll out certain improvements, be that as it may. Rather than universally handy white flour, I utilized a blend of almond and coconut flour.

I mix these two flours together constantly for Keto recipes. The almond flour is an extraordinary wellspring of fat, with irrelevant carbs.

Coconut flour offers a lighter surface. You'll see there is considerably less coconut flour than almond flour utilized in this formula.

That is because coconut flour absorbs fluid like a wipe and extends. A little goes far.

Different Ingredients

Likewise present in these bagels in a lesser sum is psyllium husk powder. Notwithstanding being an incredible wellspring of fiber, psyllium husk pastes everything together like gluten does. I included preparing powder and a touch of vinegar to enable these bagels to rise. Garlic powder and ghee include season.

As a finale, I brush the bagels with olive oil and spread them with sesame seeds. It's flawlessness!

More Keto Diet Recipes

As this formula demonstrates, you don't need to surrender bagels and diet everlastingly because you're pursuing ketosis.

More Keto Breakfast Options

A great many people like bagels toward the beginning of the day (except if you're one of my long distance race running companions and you eat them always), so you may be searching for different alternatives for your morning dinner.

I guarantee that there are numerous choices out there! If you're as yet wary, this book will show you the wide assortment of breakfast nourishments you can appreciate that are Keto and tasty.

INGREDIENTS

1 cup (120 g) of almond flour

1/4 cup (28 g) of coconut flour

1 Tablespoon (7 g) of psyllium husk powder

1 teaspoon (2 g) of preparing powder

1 teaspoon (3 g) of garlic powder

squeeze salt

2 medium eggs (88 g)

2 teaspoons (10 ml) of white wine vinegar

2 1/2 Tablespoons (38 ml) of ghee, liquefied

1 Tablespoon (15 ml) of olive oil
1 teaspoon (5 g) of sesame seeds
INSTRUCTIONS
Preheat the stove to 320°F (160°C).
Consolidate the almond flour, coconut flour, psyllium husk powder, heating powder, garlic powder and salt in a bowl.
In a different bowl, whisk the eggs and vinegar together. Gradually shower in the softened ghee (which ought not be sizzling) and rush in well.
Add the wet blend to the dry blend and utilize a wooden spoon to consolidate well. Leave to sit for 2-3 minutes.
Partition the blend into 4 equivalent measured segments. Utilizing your hands, shape the blend into a round shape and spot onto a plate fixed with material paper. Utilize a little spoon or apple corer to make the inside opening.
Brush the tops with olive oil and disperse over the sesame seeds. Heat in the stove for 20-25 minutes until cooked through. Permit to cool marginally before getting a charge out of!

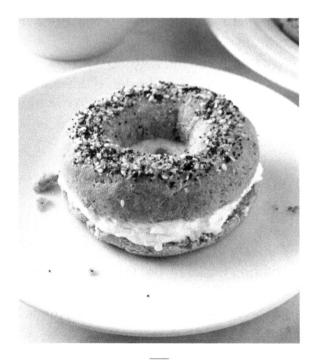

KETO BREAKFAST PIZZA

While this formula incorporates breakfast garnishes like smoked salmon and eggs, you can utilize the keto diet base for flavorful pizzas also. Utilizing a mix of riced cauliflower, coconut flour, and psyllium husk, this formula holds up well to even the heaviest pizza garnishes. In addition, each filling serving runs you 7 net carbs.

What's better time than pizza for breakfast? This low-carb breakfast pizza is made totally without any preparation from beginning to end in under 25 minutes. Since the outside layer blends and cooks so rapidly, it's ideal for mornings where you need an extravagant breakfast without a huge amount of exertion.

When your morning meal pizza outside is cooked and prepared, it's the ideal opportunity for garnishes. I beat my morning meal pizza with smoked salmon, avocado, new herbs, sauteed spinach, and a sprinkle of olive oil. Yet, pizza limits are intended to be broken, so get inventive! Attempt bacon and eggs, the previous evening's scraps, chimichurri sauce, broiled veggies, or kimchi or sauerkraut.

Have pizza for breakfast: This keto-accommodating breakfast pizza controls your morning with quality fat and fiber in less than 30 minutes. Paleo and Whole30.

KETO BREAKFAST PIZZA

All the way: 25 minutes

INGREDIENTS:

2 cups ground cauliflower

2 tablespoons coconut flour

1/2 teaspoon salt

4 eggs

1 tablespoon psyllium husk powder (Use a shape free brand like this one)

Garnishes: smoked Salmon, avocado, herbs, spinach, olive oil (see post for more recommendations)

Cushioned Keto Almond Flour Biscuits

16 Diner-Worthy Keto Shake Recipes With Zero Added Sugar

Firm Keto Cauliflower Tots

Keto Pavlova Recipe

INSTRUCTIONS:

Preheat the stove to 350 degrees. Line a pizza plate or sheet container with material.

In a blending bowl, include all ingredients with the exception of fixings and blend until joined. Put in a safe spot for 5 minutes to permit coconut flour and psyllium husk to retain fluid and thicken up.

Cautiously pour the morning meal pizza base onto the container. Utilize your hands to form it into a round, even pizza outside layer.

Prepare for 15 minutes, or until brilliant dark colored and completely cooked.

Expel from the stove and top breakfast pizza with your picked garnishes. Serve warm.

Serves: 2

BREAKFAST PIZZA NUTRITIONAL INFORMATION (PER SERVING):

Calories: 454

Complete Fat: 31g

Soaked Fat: 75g

Cholesterol: 348mg

Complete Carbs: 26g

Fiber: 17.2g

Sugars: 4.4g

Net Carbs: 8.8g

Protein: 22g

Sodium: 1,325mg

Potassium: 991mg

Calcium: 235mg

Nutrient D: 35mcg

Iron: 3mg

BREAKFAST PIZZA NUTRITIONAL INFORMATION (PER SERVING, CRUST ONLY):

Calories: 226

Complete Fat: 11g

Soaked Fat: 55g

Cholesterol: 327mg

Sodium: 765mg

Complete Carbs: 18g

Fiber: 11g

Complete Sugars: 4.1g

Net Carbs: 7g

Protein: 15g

Nutrient D: 31mcg

Calcium: 204mg

Iron: 2mg

Potassium: 421mg

Note on ingredients: Heavy strands like psyllium husk can sit undigested in our guts, sustaining awful microorganisms. In enormous sums, it can likewise cause GI trouble. Utilize great psyllium husk whenever conceivable, devour just once in a while, and get a greater amount of your fiber from entire vegetables.

COCONUT FLOUR PIZZA CRUST

Make this keto diet pizza base firm and thin, or fold it into a thicker, fluffier outside — regardless of how you set it up, this formula removes all dairy, grains, and gluten for a sum of 6 net carbs. Coconut flour and psyllium makes a firm surface, while apple juice vinegar loans a tart flavor.

A pizza hull made of coconut flour that is so natural to get ready and delightful to eat. This coconut flour pizza covering can be made into either a flimsy fresh outside layer, or a thicker cushy hull. It is totally without gluten, sans grain, low-carb and ketogenic. It can without much of a stretch be adjusted for Paleo and sans dairy too.

A pizza covering made of coconut flour that is so natural to get ready and scrumptious to eat. This coconut flour pizza outside layer can be made into either a dainty fresh hull, or a thicker soft covering. It is totally without gluten, sans grain, low-carb and ketogenic. It can without much of a stretch be adjusted for Paleo and sans dairy too.

I have attempted many pizza outsides in the previous eighteen months on my gluten and sans grain venture. There are some that ended up alright, and others that turned out and out horrendous.

Some I even needed to eat with a spoon, because there had no possibility of lifting them up with your hand effectively. And afterward extremely, what's the purpose of making a pizza if it requires a spoon? That is increasingly similar to a pizza mush.

After a lot of experimentation, I at last found this coconut flour pizza covering which is a very delicious and pickupable (truly, I incidentally make up my very own words) outside that can be made either into a thick, or a dainty hull. It is absolutely equipped for being grabbed and holding together, regardless of whether you load a huge amount of garnishes on there.

A pizza hull made of coconut flour that is so natural to get ready and delightful to eat. This coconut flour pizza outside layer can be made into either a flimsy firm covering, or a thicker fleecy hull. It is totally sans gluten, sans grain, low-carb and ketogenic. It can undoubtedly be adjusted for Paleo and without dairy also. The thick covering is overly cushioned and the meager outside layer is decent and firm. It truly works incredible for the two kinds. In spite of the fact that, I should state that I am a slender and fresh sort of individual myself.

To make these delightful pizza outsides, you'll need to begin by expelling the bunches from your coconut flour. You can do this by sifting it, or by setting it in a bowl and squashing with a fork until the entirety of the lumps are no more.

To the bowl, include your psyllium husk powder (more on this in a minute), garlic powder and salt, and blend until consolidated. Next, you'll need to include your apple juice vinegar, heating pop and eggs. Combine that all until completely joined.

A pizza outside made of coconut flour that is so natural to get ready and tasty to eat. This coconut flour pizza covering can be made into either a slight firm outside layer, or a thicker fleecy hull. It is totally without gluten, sans grain, low-carb and ketogenic. It can without much of a stretch be adjusted for Paleo and sans dairy too. Include some bubbling water and blend well. If the batter is excessively clingy, include more coconut flour, however don't include excessively. You may need to utilize the back of a spoon or wet fingers to smooth out the batter onto a preparing sheet, because it is somewhat clingy paying little respect to the consistency.

Spread on a preparing sheet with material paper, or my top choice, a silicone heating mat, to your ideal thickness (it will lighten up a piece, however not significantly), and fly in the stove for 15-20 minutes, or until it starts to dark colored around the edges. Expel from broiler and top with your ideal ingredients. Spot back in the broiler until the cheddar is softened, and you're altogether done!

A pizza outside layer made of coconut flour that is so natural to plan and delightful to eat. This coconut flour pizza outside layer can be made into either a meager firm covering, or a thicker soft hull. It is totally without gluten, sans grain, low-carb and ketogenic. It can without much of a stretch be adjusted for Paleo and sans dairy too.

Psyllium husk powder is a type of fiber that assimilates dampness and tie the outside layer together. I find that is gives low-carb and sans gluten prepared products a more diet-like surface. It is extraordinary for your absorption and can help move things along if you need assistance around there.

When psyllium husk powder and high temp water are joined, the psyllium husk frames a thick surface that goes about as a paste to tie the outside layer together. In any case, don't stress over this covering being thick, when it is warmed, the fluid vanishes and structures a decent firm outside layer. These coconut flour supper rolls likewise incorporate the marvelousness that is psyllium husk powder!

A pizza outside layer made of coconut flour that is so natural to get ready and flavorful to eat. This coconut flour pizza outside layer can be made into either a flimsy fresh covering, or a thicker cushy hull. It is totally without gluten, sans grain, low-carb and ketogenic. It can without much of a stretch be adjusted for Paleo and sans dairy too.

I trust all of you appreciated this delectable coconut flour pizza outside. It was a work of affection to make, and one I trust you folks all appreciate eating. If you give it a shot, let me comprehend what you think in the remarks beneath! If you delighted in this formula, I think you'd likewise like a portion of the other Italian dishes I bring to the table.

Likewise, if you delighted in this formula, you will LOVE this two-fixing skillet pizza covering! I guarantee ☺

A pizza outside layer made of coconut flour that is so natural to plan and heavenly to eat. This coconut flour pizza covering can be made into either a slight fresh outside layer, or a thicker fleecy hull. It is totally sans gluten, without grain, low-carb and ketogenic. It can without much of a stretch be adjusted for Paleo and sans dairy also.

Coconut Flour Pizza Crust

A pizza outside layer made of coconut flour that is so natural to plan and heavenly to eat. This coconut flour pizza outside layer can be made into either a flimsy fresh covering, or a thicker cushioned hull. It is totally sans gluten, without grain, low-carb and ketogenic. It can without much of a stretch be adjusted for Paleo and sans dairy also.

INGREDIENTS

3/4 cup coconut flour bunches expelled

3 tablespoons psyllium husk powder

1 teaspoon garlic powder

1/2 teaspoon Salt I love this Himalayan pink salt

1 teaspoon apple juice vinegar

1/2 teaspoon heating pop

3 eggs

1 cup bubbling water

A pizza outside layer made of coconut flour that is so natural to get ready and scrumptious to eat. This coconut flour pizza outside can be made into either a dainty firm covering, or a thicker cushy hull. It is totally without gluten, sans grain, low-carb and ketogenic. It can without much of a stretch be adjusted for Paleo and sans dairy also.

INSTRUCTIONS

Preheat broiler to 350F.

Blend coconut flour with psyllium husk powder, garlic powder and salt until completely consolidated.

Include apple juice vinegar, heating pop and eggs. Combine.

Blend bubbling water in, and mix until joined. If the mixture is excessively clingy, include more coconut flour until it is the ideal consistency. The batter will normally be somewhat clingy however, so you might need to utilize wet fingers to spread out the mixture.

Spread mixture out on a preparing sheet to the ideal thickness. I like mine to be quite dainty, so my mixture as a rule covers the whole preparing sheet.

Spot in a preheated broiler for 15-20 minutes, or until edges start to dark colored.

Top with sauce, cheddar and wanted fixings and spot back in the stove until the cheddar is dissolved.

CHOCOLATE CHAFFLE

At this point, you have presumably known about the chaffle. It is the best in class keto development, and in light of current circumstances!

Chaffles are typically a mix of cheddar and egg, now and then blended in with other heating specialists like preparing powder, however this is the no frills, fundamental form of the chaffle. To see this variant of a chaffle, see our Easy Traditional Keto Chaffle Recipe.

There is a lot more you can do with a chaffle than simply making it with cheddar and egg! There are breakfast chaffles, sandwich chaffles, and even treat chaffles, similar to this one! Obviously, there are slight varieties relying upon what sort of keto chaffle you are making.

Keto Chocolate Chaffle Ingredients

1 egg
1 oz cream cheddar
2 tablespoons almond flour
1 tablespoon unsweetened cocoa powder
2 teaspoons priest organic product
1 teaspoon vanilla concentrate
Keto Chocolate Chaffle Directions
1 Preheat waffle producer to medium high warmth.
2 Whisk together egg, cream cheddar, almond flour, cocoa powder, priest organic product, and vanilla.
3 Pour chaffle blend into the focal point of the waffle iron. Close the waffle producer and let cook for 3-5 minutes or until waffle is brilliant dark colored and set.
4 Remove chaffle from the waffle creator and serve.

LOW CARB CHOCOLATE CHAFFLE RECIPE

A chaffle is a keto agreeable waffle that is principally comprised of cheddar and egg. That is the reason it's known as a chaffle. Chocolate chaffles make the perfect breakfast when you need something sweet or immaculate pastry when you have a chocolate desiring up don't have any desire to disturb the problem of making a keto dessert with loads of steps and fixings. Chocolate chaffles can be made under 5 minutes.

Swerve can be utilized rather than Lakanto Monkfruit, and the estimation is the equivalent.

Fixings

1 egg

1 tbsp substantial whipping cream

1/2 tsp coconut flour

1 3/4 tsp Lakanto monkfruit brilliant can utilize pretty much to change sweetness

1/4 tsp heating powder

spot of salt

1 tbsp Lily's Chocolate Chips

Guidelines

Turn on the waffle producer so it warms up.

In a little bowl, join all fixings aside from the chocolate chips and mix well until consolidated.

Oil waffle producer, then pour half of the player onto the base plate of the waffle creator. Sprinkle a couple of chocolate chips on top and afterward close.

Cook for 3-4 minutes or until the chocolate chip chaffle sweet is brilliant dark colored then expel from waffle creator with a fork, being mindful so as not to consume your fingers.

PUMPKIN CHOCOLATE CHIP CHAFFLES

When fall comes I start hauling out all that I can that includes pumpkin. Pumpkin Chocolate Chip flapjacks have consistently been my preferred pumpkin breakfast, with a salted caramel pumpkin latte. I thought without a doubt this year I would need to skip it again like a year ago.

I took a stab at making pumpkin chocolate chip treats that were low carb however they were a failure. I attempted so often that I surrendered. It may be because I am fastidious with the surfaces and flavors that accompany a pumpkin anything.

So was the pumpkin chocolate chip flapjacks I attempted to make. This year when the chaffle furor began in the wake of making bunches of different chaffles and concocting new chaffle plans, I realized that it was the ideal time for me to make a pumpkin chocolate chip chaffle.

I thought of these pumpkin chocolate chip chaffles and they are delish! I like them beat with swerve confectioners or keto whipped cream!

For this pumpkin chaffle we're utilizing mozzarella cheddar which totally vanishes and includes no cheddar enhance! You truly won't know it's in there – simply trust me.

Fixings

1/2 cup destroyed mozzarella cheddar

4 teaspoons pumpkin puree

1 egg

2 tablespoons granulated swerve

1/4 tsp pumpkin pie flavor

4 teaspoons sugar free chocolate chips

1 tablespoon almond flour

Directions

Plug in your waffle creator.

In a little bowl blend the pumpkin puree and egg. Ensure you blend it well so all the pumpkin is blended in with the egg.

Next include the mozzarella cheddar, almond flour, swerve and pumpkin flavor and blend well.

Then include your sugar free chocolate chips

Include a large portion of the keto pumpkin pie Chaffle blend to the Dish Mini waffle creator at once. Cook chaffle player in the waffle creator for 4 minutes.

Try not to open before the 4 minutes is up. It is VERY significant that you don't open the waffle creator before the brief imprint. After that you can open it to check it and ensure it is cooked the whole distance, yet with these chaffles keeping the top shut the entire time is VERY significant.

When the first is totally done cooking cook the subsequent one. Appreciate with some swerve confectioners' sugar or whipped cream on top.

Nourishment

Serving: 1g | Calories: 93kcal | Carbohydrates: 2g | Protein: 7g | Fat: 7g | Saturated Fat: 3g | Cholesterol: 69mg | Sodium: 138mg | Potassium: 48mg | Fiber: 1g | Sugar: 1g | Vitamin A: 1228IU | Calcium: 107mg | Iron: 1mg

MINT CHOCOLATE CHAFFLE

Fundamental, BEST CHAFFLE RECIPE
1 egg, beaten
1/2 cup cheddar
Layer 1/8 cup of cheddar on the base of the waffle producer.
Include a large portion of the beaten egg.
Layer the other 1/8 cup of cheddar on top.
Cook until fresh. Remember the chaffle gets crispier as it cools.
Chaffles are extremely popular because despite the fact that I have a huge amount of Keto bread plans like my Keto Bread, Keto Cheese Muffins, Keto Blueberry Muffins, Cauliflower breadsticks, and Keto Pancakes – at times individuals need something bready that they can make instantly

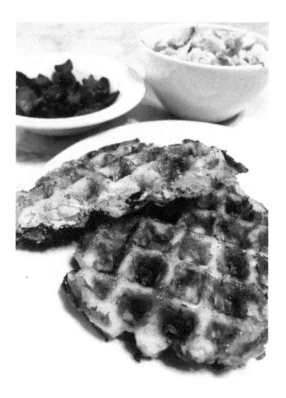

APPETIZING CHAFFLE RECIPES

Everything except for THE BAGEL CHAFFLE RECIPE
Utilize the base formula
Include Everything except the Bagel Seasoning to taste. – Julia A.
RICH and CREAMY CHAFFLES RECIPE
2 eggs
1 cup destroyed mozzarella
2 tablespoons almond flour
2 tablespoons cream cheddar
3/4 teaspoon preparing power
3 tablespoons water (discretionary)
Combine all fixings.
Cook in a smaller than normal waffle iron for 4 minutes, or until firm.
Makes 6 waffles. – Shelly J.

ZUCCHINI CHUFFLES | ZUFFLES RECIPE

1 little zucchini, ground
1 egg
1 tablespoon parmesan
Little bunch of destroyed mozzarella
Basil and pepper to taste
Combine all and cook in a full size waffle creator.
Makes 2 full size zaffles and a scanty zaffle. – Marian R.

LIGHT and CRISPY CHAFFLES RECIPE

1 egg
1/3 cup cheddar
1/4 teaspoon heating powder
1/2 teaspoon ground flaxseed
Destroyed parmesan cheddar on top and base.
Blend and cook in a smaller than expected waffle iron until fresh. – Kim H.

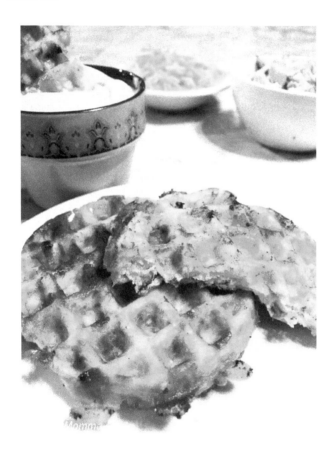

BACON CHEDDAR CHAFFLES RECIPE

1 egg
1.2 cup cheddar
Bacon bits to taste
Blend and cook until fresh. – Jennifer H.
BACON JALAPENO CHAFFLES RECIPE
1/2 cup destroyed swiss/gruyere mix
1 egg
2 tablespoons cooked bacon pieces
1 tablespoon diced crisp jalapenos
Cook until fresh. Works incredible as a bun to a cheeseburger. – Meagan J.

EXQUISITE CAULIFLOWER CHAFFLES

This formula is mine. Look at this formula to make simple, 15-minute cauliflower chaffles. They'd make a spectacular cauliflower pizza outside for you also!

SANDWICH BREAD CHAFFLES RECIPE

1 egg

2 tablespoon almond flour

1 tablespoon mayo

1/8 teaspoon heating powder

1 teaspoon water

Sugar and garlic powder (discretionary)

Makes 2 chaffles, and you can without much of a stretch cut them down the middle for a bun. – Linda K.

LEMON POUND CAKE CHAFFLES

Numerous individuals are cutting my lemon pound cake formula by 1/4 and making Cake Chaffles out of them.

Crusty fruit-filled treat CHAFFLES

1.2 cup mozzarella cheddar

1 egg

Add the mozzarella to the waffle producer.

Put the egg on top.

Sprinkle on crusty fruit-filled treat zest and 5 sugar free chocolate chips.

Present with margarine on top. – Stacy G.

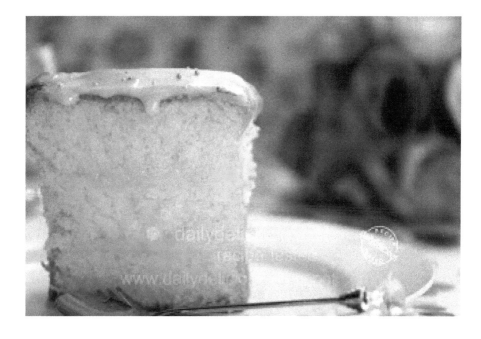

CREAM CHEESE CARROT CAKE CHAFFLES

2 tablespoons cream cheddar or a blend of 1 tablespoon cream cheddar and 2 tablespoons destroyed mozzarella cheddar
1/2 pat of margarine
1 tablespoon finely destroyed carrot
1 tablespoon of sugar of your decision. I utilized Splenda.
1 tablespoon almond flour
1 teaspoon pumpkin pie zest
1/2 teaspoon vanilla
1/2 teaspoon heating powder
1 egg
Discretionary
I included 6 raisins, 1 tablespoon of destroyed coconut and 1/2 tablespoon of pecans to the blender fixings.

CREAM CHEESE FROSTING

1 tablespoon cream cheddar

1 pat margarine

1 teaspoon sugar of decision. I utilized Cinnamon Brown Sugar sans sugar syrup.

Warmth up waffle producer. I utilized a smaller than usual Dash. I oiled with a silicon brush plunged in coconut oil.

Microwave cream cheddar, mozzarella, and margarine for 15 seconds to dissolve the cheeses to make joining simpler. I did this in an enchantment shot cup to mix.

Include the remainder of the chaffle fixings to blender cup and mix until smooth and fused.

Add hitter to waffle producer. For the Dash, I included 2 stacking tablespoons and it made 3 chaffles.

While making the chaffle, heat up the margarine and cream cheddar for the icing. Blend until smooth and fuse your sugar. Shower over chaffles as wanted. – Heather S.

CINNAMON CHAFFLES

1/2 cup mozzarella
1 egg
1 tbsp vanilla concentrate
1/2 tsp preparing powder
1 tbsp almond flour
Sprinkle of cinnamon
Combine and cook until chaffles are firm.

CINNAMON SWIRL CHAFFLES

CHAFFLE:
1 oz cream cheddar, softened
1 huge egg, beaten
1 tsp vanilla concentrate
1 tbsp almond flour, superfine
1 tbsp Splenda
1 tsp cinnamon
ICING:
1 oz cream cheddar, softened
1 tbsp margarine, unsalted
1 tbsp Splenda
1/2 tsp vanilla
CINNAMON DRIZZLE:
1/2 tbsp margarine
1 tbsp Splenda
1 tsp cinnamon
Warmth up waffle producer, I brushed on coconut oil on my DASH.
Stir up the chaffle fixings until smooth.
Utilize a spoon to include 2 storing tbsp of hitter to the waffle iron. It will make 3 little waffles.
Cook to your ideal waffle freshness. I did 4 min, they resembled a delicate waffle.
Cool on a rack.
Blend the icing and cinnamon sprinkle in little bowls. Warmth in microwave for 10 secs to get to a delicate consistency. Twirl on cooled waffles.
Fixings
1 Cup (235mL) Heavy Cream
1/4 Tsp Peppermint Extract
1 Heaping Tbsp (8g) Keto Chocolate Chips – 0 NET CARBS
Only under 3 Tbsps (24g) Confectioners Swerve
1/8 Tsp (3 Drops) Green Food Coloring

Directions

On a cutting barricade slash the keto chocolate chips.

Presently, include the entirety of the fixings (sparing portion of the keto chocolate chips for some other time) to a widemouth bricklayer container at any rate 16oz huge.

Shake enthusiastically for a few minutes.

When the overwhelming cream begins to thicken up – and nearly duplicates in size – include the remainder of the keto chocolate chips and shake once more.

Freeze for 4-5 hours, or until strong

*If freezing for longer than 5 hours use Allulose rather than Confectioners Swerve to prevent the frozen yogurt from freezing strong

Mint Chocolate Chip Mason Jar Keto Ice Cream

KETO WHIPPED CREAM

Whipped cream is very simple to make thus much better for you and the earth than the prepackaged stuff. You won't ever need to return to the airborne form once you make this..
Fixings
Dry Ingredients
1/4 Cup Almond Flour.
1 Tbsp. Cocoa Powder (unsweetened)
1-1/2 Tbsp. Erythritol
½ tsp heating powder
Wet Ingredients
1 Large Egg.
2 Tbsp Butter or coconut oil. softened
1/2 tsp Vanilla Extract discretionary
1/4 cup almond milk (unsweetened)

Guidelines

Preheat waffle iron while you are blending the fixings.
soften spread in microwave
In a little blending bowl blend all the dry fixings. Ensure there are no bunches
Include egg, softened spread, almond milk, and utilize an elastic scrubber to blend altogether.
pour the blend in the focal point of lubed waffle iron waffle iron and close. (flip it if you have on of those extravagant Belgian waffle irons)
Cook until wanted freshness. I normally set a clock for 10 minutes.
Open the waffle iron, expel and appreciate.

Notes

Coconut oil will just take around ten seconds to dissolve in the microwave.

BROWNIE BATTER

I've been utilizing These No Sugar Chocolate Chips From Lily's for a long, long time. They're totally delightful and just have 2 NET CARBS. Also, you can get them on Amazon, or even discover them in your nearby market!

Nonetheless, Lily's simply turned out with a 0 NET CARB Semi-Sweetened Chocolate Chip that is far and away superior to those!

I know, it doesn't bode well, however I don't make the chocolate chips, I simply eat them. Also, I can let you know unquestionably, the new form is mind-blowingly great.

The main issue for me is that they're not on Amazon right now. What's more, I haven't seen them in my supermarket either.

Ideally, they'll be simpler to get soon.

In any case, I exceptionally urge you to utilize them for your keto brownie hitter!

Fixings

Loading Tbsp (17g) Salted Butter
2 Tbsps (25g) No Sugar Chocolate Chips
A little more than 1/3 Cup (40g) Kirkland's Blanched Almond Flour
2 Tbsps (20g) Confectioners Swerve
Loading Tbsp (6g) Unsweetened Cocoa Powder
1/4 Tsp Pure Vanilla Extract
Touch of Salt
2 Tbsps (25g) Unsweetened Vanilla Almond Milk

Directions

Cut up the spread into little squares and add them to a medium-sized bowl

Next, include the chocolate chips and microwave for 20-30 seconds (or until the spread melts)

When the spread has dissolved, utilize a spatula to join it with the chocolate chips

---

When the spread and chocolate chips have joined to shape a "chocolate sauce" include the remainder of the fixings
Presently utilize a spatula to work the fixings into each other until a player creates
Appreciate

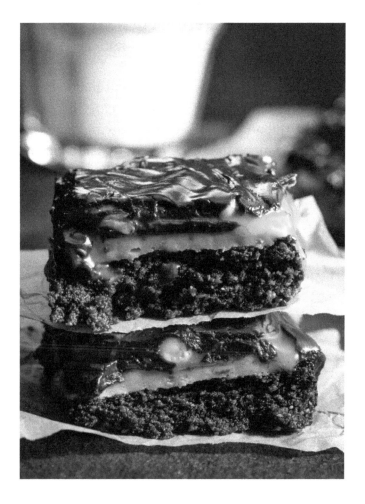

KETO CRISPY CHOCO CHAFFLE

Since chaffles have taken the low-carb/keto world by storm, I thought it'd be great to share our essential Crispy Keto Chaffle formula with every one of our guests! There are numerous varieties of the chaffle, however this is the straightforward adaptation we use when we're searching for a toasted bread substitution.

Presently if you're prepared, we should chaffle!

Preparing Time 1M

Cooking Time 6M

All out Time 7M

Net Carb/Waffle ~1g

Servings 2 Waffles

Fixings

1 Egg

1/2 Cup Shredded Cheese

Headings

1) Gather every one of the fixings.

2) Plug-in Dash Mini Waffle Maker to pre-heat.

Keto Cauli Chicken Chaffle Recipe

3) In a little blending bowl, beat egg.

4) Place around 1/8 cup destroyed cheddar on to the Dash Mini Waffle Maker, trailed by ~1/2 of the egg blend (enough to cover the iron) and another 1/8 cup of destroyed cheddar on top. Close top and cook for 3 – 4 minutes. Rehash for the same number of waffles you are making.

5) Let the chaffle cool for a couple of moments before gathering your preferred sandwich.

Firm Keto Chaffle Recipe (8)

Expectation you make the most of your low-carb/keto Crispy Keto Chaffle !

Chaffles are cheddar + waffles = chaffles! Fun, isn't that so?

CHAFFLES NUTRITION INFO AND CARB COUNT

The calories and carbs in chaffles will differ contingent upon the rendition you make and what you put in them. The following is the sustenance data for all the different renditions I made for you.

TIP: The sustenance information recorded is consistently for 1 smaller than normal chaffle (for simple scaling), yet once in a while you could have two, for example, for a sandwich or full supper. The fundamental chaffle and garlic Parmesan plans make 2 scaled down chaffles each. The cinnamon sugar (churro), pumpkin, and zesty jalapeno popper plans make 3 scaled down chaffles each.

Essential CHAFFLE RECIPE FOR SANDWICHES:

These are out and out chaffles! They are really unbiased, not sweet or appetizing, making them extraordinary for sandwiches.

208 calories

2g net carbs

16g fat

11g protein

GARLIC PARMESAN CHAFFLES:

These resemble garlic bread in chaffle structure. I like fixing them with extra softened mozzarella, ground parmesan, and a pinch of parsley.

182 calories

2g net carbs

11g fat

16g protein

CINNAMON SUGAR (CHURRO) CHAFFLES:

Who doesn't cherish churros?! You can eat these chaffles entire, or for a more churro-like understanding, cut them into sticks.

179 calories

2g net carbs

14g fat

10g protein

PUMPKIN CHAFFLES:

I like to utilize hand crafted pumpkin pie zest for these, however locally acquired fills in also. A dab of whipped cream and a sprinkle of cinnamon makes them simply great.

117 calories

3g net carbs

7g fat

7g protein

Fiery JALAPENO POPPER CHAFFLES:

Huge numbers of you have approached me for hot chaffles, so I made these jalapeno popper enhanced ones! Softened cheddar, bacon bits, and a couple jalapeno cuts make the ideal garnish.

231 calories

2g net carbs

18g fat

13g protein

CHAFFLE RECIPE FOR SANDWICHES:

1/2 cup Mozzarella cheddar (destroyed)
1 enormous Egg
2 tbsp Blanched almond flour (or 2 tsp coconut flour)
1/2 tsp Psyllium husk powder (discretionary, however prescribed for surface, sprinkle in so it doesn't bunch)
1/4 tsp Baking powder (discretionary)
Garlic Parmesan Chaffles:
1/2 cup Mozzarella cheddar (destroyed)
1/3 cup Grated Parmesan cheddar
1 enormous Egg
1 clove Garlic (minced; or utilize 1/2 clove for milder garlic enhance)
1/2 tsp Italian flavoring
1/4 tsp Baking powder (discretionary)
Cinnamon Sugar (Churro) Chaffles:
1 enormous Egg
3/4 cup Mozzarella cheddar (destroyed)
2 tbsp Blanched almond flour (or 2 tsp coconut flour)
1/2 tbsp Butter (liquefied)
2 tbsp Erythritol
1/2 tsp Cinnamon
1/2 tsp Vanilla concentrate
1/2 tsp Psyllium husk powder (discretionary, for surface)
1/4 tsp Baking powder (discretionary)
1 tbsp Butter (liquefied; for fixing)
1/4 cup Erythritol (for fixing)
3/4 tsp Cinnamon (for garnish)
Pumpkin Chaffles:
1/2 oz Cream cheddar
1 enormous Egg
1/2 cup Mozzarella cheddar (destroyed)
2 tbsp Pumpkin puree
2 1/2 tbsp Erythritol

---

3 tsp Coconut flour

1/2 tbsp Pumpkin pie zest

1/2 tsp Vanilla concentrate (discretionary)

1/4 tsp Baking powder (discretionary)

Zesty Jalapeno Popper Chaffles:

1 oz Cream cheddar

1 enormous Egg

1 cup cheddar (destroyed)

2 tbsp Bacon bits

1/2 tbsp Jalapenos

1/4 tsp Baking powder (discretionary)

Guidelines

Formula TIPS + VIDEO in the post above, sustenance data + formula notes beneath!

Snap on the occasions in the guidelines beneath to begin a kitchen clock while you cook.

Guidelines:

Preheat your waffle iron for around 5 minutes, until hot.

If the formula contains cream cheddar, place it into a bowl first. Warmth it delicately in the microwave (~15-30 seconds) or a twofold heater, until it's delicate and simple to mix.

Mix in all other residual fixings (with the exception of garnishes, if any).

Pour enough of the chaffle player into the waffle producer to cover the surface well. (That is around 1/2 cup player for a customary waffle producer and 1/4 cup for a smaller than expected waffle creator.)

Cook until carmelized and fresh, around 3-4 minutes. (See my tip in the post above about different approaches to tell they are managed without opening the waffle producer!)

Cautiously expel the chaffle from the waffle producer and put aside to fresh up additional. (Cooling is significant for surface!)

Repeat with outstanding player, if any.

Uncommon guidance for churro chaffles as it were:

Mix together the erythritol and cinnamon for garnish. After the chaffles are cooked and no longer hot, brush them with liquefied spread, then sprinkle done with the cinnamon "sugar" garnish (or plunge into the fixing).

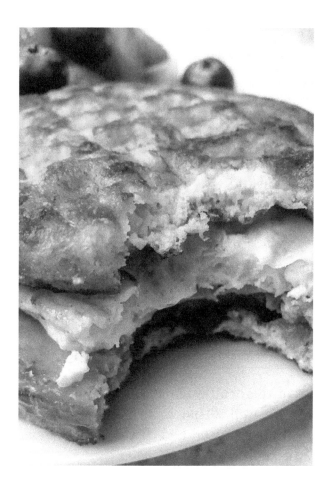

KETO PIZZA CHAFFLE

Best Keto Pizza Chaffle Recipe
The chaffle has overwhelmed the keto world, and which is all well and good, as it opens a universe of potential outcomes for those following a ketogenic diet to appreciate bread that is exceptionally low carb. There are a wide range of varieties to the conventional chaffle formula. I've had a ton of fun evaluating different plans that my kitchen has resembled a debacle. Since pizza is one of my preferred nourishments when I saw the first chaffle post, I knew a keto pizza chaffle formula would be at the highest priority on my rundown to make.

Fixings
1 tsp coconut flour
1 egg white
1/2 cup mozzarella cheddar, destroyed
'1 tsp cream cheddar, softened
1/4 tsp preparing powder
1/8 tsp Italian flavoring
1/8 tsp garlic powder
touch of salt
3 tsp low carb marinara sauce
1/2 cup mozzarella cheddar
6 pepperonis cut down the middle
1 tbsp parmesan cheddar, destroyed
1/4 tsp basil flavoring

Directions
Preheat stove to 400 degrees. Turn waffle creator on or plug it in with the goal that it gets hot.
In a little bowl include coconut flour, egg white, mozzarella cheddar, softened cream cheddar, preparing powder, garlic powder, Italian seasonings, and a touch of salt.
Pour 1/2 of the hitter in the waffle creator, close the top, and cook for 3-4 minutes or until chaffle arrives at wanted doneness.

Cautiously expel chaffle from the waffle creator, then adhere to similar directions to make the second chaffle.

Top each chaffle with tomato sauce (I utilized 1/2 tsp per), pepperoni, mozzarella cheddar, and parmesan cheddar.

Spot in the broiler on a preparing sheet (or straight on the heating rack) on the first rate of the stove for 5-6 minutes. Then turn the broiler to sear with the goal that the cheddar starts to air pocket and dark colored. Keep a nearby eye as it can consume rapidly. I cooked my pizza chaffle for approx 1 min and 30 seconds.

Expel from broiler and sprinkle basil on top.

Appreciate!

Notes

The wholesome data gave is to one of the keto Pizza Chaffels with the goal that every individual could pick the amount they needed to eat to accommodate their appetite levels and health objectives.

DELICIOUS PIZZA CHAFFLE RECIPE

Heavenly KETO PIZZA CHAFFLE RECIPE
There are a few things that are simply too great to even consider giving up, and pizza is one of them. Pizza isn't actually low carb (and I mean it is brimming with carbs) which makes it difficult to eat while remaining in ketosis. There are a lot of work arounds to this issue however, similar to our Tasty Keto Pizza With Homemade Sauce.
This keto pizza chaffle formula likewise happens to be one of those work arounds, and it is as of now our most loved keto pizza! If you like the smash of a decent slender hull pizza (or even the mash of an all-around done profound dish) you will LOVE this keto chaffle pizza! It sincerely tastes precisely like you're eating the pizza you know and love from your pre-keto days.
Fixings
CHAFFLE CRUST
1 Egg
1/2 cup Mozzarella Cheese
1 tsp Coconut Flour
1/4 tsp Baking Powder
1/8 tsp Garlic Powder
1/8 tsp Italian Seasoning
Touch of Salt
PIZZA TOPPING
1 tbsp Rao's Marinara Sauce
1/2 cup Mozzarella Cheese
3 Pepperoni's, cut into four
Destroyed Parmesan Cheese, discretionary
Parsley, discretionary
Directions
Preheat stove to 400 degrees. Preheat waffle producer also.
In a little bowl, consolidate egg, mozzarella cheddar, coconut flour, heating powder, garlic powder, italian flavoring, and salt.

87

Pour half of the chaffle blend into the focal point of the waffle iron. Permit to cook for 3-5 minutres.
Cautiously evacuate and rehash for second chaffle.
Top each chaffle with sauce, mozzarella cheddar, and pepperoni.
Spot chaffles on a heating sheet and spot in the broiler for 4-5 minutes and sear for 1 moment a short time later.
Evacuate and sprinkle some parsley or basil if wanted. Appreciate

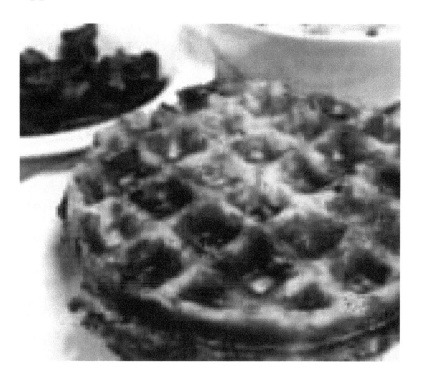

SPICY PIZZA CHAFFLE

WHAT IS A "KETO CHAFFLE PIZZA"?
You might be staying there speculation, "what on the planet is a chaffle pizza?" and trust me, I was in that spot with you half a month back. For reasons unknown, a chaffle is cheddar waffle, just it doesn't have flour in it. State what? No big surprise this is so Keto inviting! I did Keto strictly for a long time and had never known about this thing. Since I have, it's everything I need to eat!

Hot KETO CHAFFLE PIZZA
Delectable formula for a chaffle pizza, ideal for those following a low carb or Keto diet.

Course Appetizer, Main Course, Snack
Food Italian
Watchword chaffle, keto, low carb, pizza
Planning Time 3 minutes
Cook Time 10 minutes
All out Time 13 minutes
Servings 1 Serving
Calories 316 kcal

Fixings
Chaffle Pizza "Mixture"
1 Large Egg
1/2 Cup Shredded Mozzarella Cheese
1/4 tsp Baking Powder
Salt to taste
Pepper to taste
Garlic Powder to taste
Red Pepper Flakes to taste
Chaffle Pizza Toppings
1/2 TBSP Rao's Pizza Sauce (2 tsp per chaffle)
6 cuts Pepperoni
Destroyed Mozzarella Cheese to taste

Guidelines

Plug in your waffle iron and shower with cooking splash if your machine requires it.

Beat your egg marginally. Include the destroyed cheddar and seasonings and blend it up.

Sprinkle a tad of cheddar on the waffle iron. If you are utilizing the smaller than normal Dash waffle iron, place half of your chaffle "batter" blend in the waffle iron and close the top.

Cook for around 5 minutes, or until your ideal freshness has been come to.

Evacuate the chaffle and put the remaining chaffle "batter" blend on the waffle iron and cook once more.

When both chaffles are cooked, place on your pizza heating dish and top with the Rao's Pizza Sauce and wanted garnishes. Cook on low for around 5-6 minutes. Make certain to watch this part cautiously so you don't consume your Spicy Keto Chaffle Pizza.

LOW CARB PIZZA CHAFFLE CUPS

Elements FOR LOW CARB PIZZA CHAFFLES:
Our keto pizza chaffle formula makes 4 smaller than expected chaffles in a DASH scaled down waffle producer
or then again 2 chaffles if you're utilizing a Belgian Waffle Maker:
2 enormous eggs
1/4 cup superfine whitened almond flour: includes structure and makes them less eggy/mushy and more bread like
3/4 teaspoon heating powder: makes them rise and extra cushy
garlic powder
Italian flavoring
1 cup destroyed cheddar (we utilize a blend of cheddar and mozzarella)
FOR THE PIZZA TOPPINGS – CHOOSE YOUR FAVORITES:
3 tablespoons your preferred tomato/marinara sauce (we use Rao's)
destroyed mozzarella cheddar
1 tablespoon ground Parmesan cheddar
5-7 smaller than normal pepperoni cuts (OR customary pepperoni cut into equal parts)
cherry tomatoes
new basil
WHAT ARE LOW CARB TOPPINGS FOR A KETO PIZZA?
Mushrooms
Hotdog
Bacon
Dark olives
Green peppers
Spinach
Hot peppers
The most effective method to MAKE CHAFFLE PIZZA:
COAT WAFFLE IRON: Lightly splash your waffle creator with cooking shower or ghee and let it heat up on high.

MAKE THE BATTER: In a blending bowl, whisk together the eggs, almond flour, garlic powder, Italian flavoring and preparing powder.

The most effective method to COOK PIZZA CHAFFLES IF USING A BELGIAN WAFFLE MAKER:
Pour half of the waffle hitter into the center of your waffle iron and close the top. Cook until firm, flip and cook again as fundamental

Instructions to MAKE PIZZA CHAFFLES IF USING A DASH MINI WAFFLE MAKER:
Pour 1/4 cup of the waffle player into the center of your waffle iron and close the cover. Cook until firm, flip and cook again as important.

SERVE HOT: Carefully move to a heating sheet and top each chaffle with tomato sauce, pepperoni, mozzarella cheddar and Parmesan cheddar. Include some other garnishes as wanted.

Spot chaffles on material lined preparing sheet and spot in a preheated broiler at 375 F and heat for 4-5 minutes, or until the cheddar starts to air pocket and darker. Top with crisp basil, if wanted.

Would you be able to HAVE PIZZA ON KETO?
Indeed! Since they're made with eggs and cheddar, they are totally grain free, gluten free, low carb and ketogenic cordial.

The dietary data for 1 smaller than usual pizza chaffle is:
216 calories
4g NET CARBS = 5g Total Carbs − 1g Fiber
17g Fat
16g Protein
1g Sugar

The most effective method to STORE PIZZA CHAFFLES:
The incredible thing about making these low carb pizza outside layers is that you can make a major clump on your dinner prep Sunday and store them in the refrigerator or cooler when you're prepared to eat them.

Would you be able to FREEZE PIZZA CHAFFLES?

Lay the chaffles level in a solitary layer on a heating sheet. Spot the container in the cooler for 30 minutes. Move to an enormous resealable cooler pack or a hermetically sealed freezable holder.
TO REHEAT LOW CARB PIZZA WAFFLES:
Evacuate the low carb pizza waffles from the cooler and warm them in the waffle producer or in the broiler at 350F until firm. Include your fixings and heat again until the cheddar has dissolved.
Fixings
2 enormous eggs
1/4 cup superfine whitened almond flour
1/2 teaspoon garlic powder
1/2 teaspoon Italian flavoring
3/4 teaspoon heating powder
1 cup destroyed cheddar (we utilize a blend of cheddar and mozzarella)
3 tablespoons marinara sauce
1/2 cup destroyed mozzarella cheddar
1 tablespoon ground Parmesan cheddar
5-7 small scale pepperoni cuts (OR ordinary pepperoni cuts, cut down the middle)
Discretionary TOPPINGS:
4-5 cherry tomatoes , cut in equal parts
1 teaspoon naturally cleaved basil
Hardware

MAPLE PUMPKIN KETO CHAFFLE

Maple Pumpkin Keto Waffle Recipe (Chaffle)
My better half cherishes everything pumpkin, so I knew when I originally observed the exceptionally famous chaffle formula, I needed to make a pumpkin chaffle only for him. Rather than making just two chaffles, this formula makes four. They are so tasty you'll need more for some other time, or for my situation, we have enough for both my hubby and myself. We had it for breakfast, however you could likewise appreciate it as a delectable sweet with a scoop of keto-accommodating frozen yogurt and walnuts on top.

Fixings
2 eggs
3/4 tsp heating powder
2 tsp pumpkin puree (100% pumpkin)
3/4 tsp pumpkin pie zest
4 tsp substantial whipping cream
2 tsp Lakanto Sugar-Free Maple Syrup
1 tsp coconut flour
1/2 cup mozzarella cheddar, destroyed
1/2 tsp vanilla
spot of salt

Guidelines
Turn on waffle or chaffle producer. I utilize the Dash Mini Waffle Maker.
In a little bowl, join all fixings.
Spread the scramble smaller than normal waffle creator with 1/4 of the player and cook for 3-4 minutes.
Rehash 3 additional occasions until you have made 4 Maple Syrup Pumpkin Keto Waffles (Chaffles).
Present with sans sugar maple syrup or keto dessert.

Notes
The sugar alcohols from the Lakanto Maple Syrup are excluded from net carbs as most subtract to compute net carbs.

—

Sustenance

Serving: 2Chaffles | Calories: 201kcal | Carbohydrates: 4g | Protein: 12g | Fat: 15g | Saturated Fat: 8g | Cholesterol: 200mg | Sodium: 249mg | Potassium: 271mg | Fiber: 1g | Sugar: 1g | Vitamin A: 1341IU | Calcium: 254mg | Iron: 1mg

KETO BREAKFAST CHAFFLE

Here's a keto breakfast sandwich formula that you can really hold! Flavorful, mushy chaffles replace bread in this curve on the custom bacon and egg breakfast sandwich.

Chaffle breakfast sandwiches are a delectable feast that will keep you cheerful and full for quite a while. This formula truly hits the spot — and will definitly substitute any longings you have for inexpensive food breakfast sandwiches.

Fixings IN CHAFFLE BREAKFAST SANDWICHES

This formula for keto breakfast sandwiches made with chaffles requires moderately not many fixings. For the chaffles themselves, you'll just need two fixings:

1 huge egg

1/2 cup of destroyed cheddar

This will make enough chaffle hitter for 2 scaled down chaffles — or the two "buns" of our morning meal sandwich.

Then, for the filling of the sandwich, you can pick between a wide range of keto-accommodating fixings. In this variant, I've utilized

thick-cut bacon

singed egg

cut cheddar

In any case, this formula would likewise be incredible with:

frankfurter

ham

fried eggs

cut avocado

sauteed mushroom and peppers

hot sauce, and so forth!

Step by step instructions to MAKE KETO BREAKFAST SANDWICHES WITH CHAFFLES

—

The main thing you'll have to do to make chaffle breakfast sandwiches is to make your chaffle "bread". Fortunately, making chaffles is so fast and simple. Through and through, it takes under 5 minutes.

A keto chaffle is a waffle produced using two fundamental fixings: egg and destroyed cheddar. For a chaffle breakfast sandwich, I like to utilize cheddar. However, you can utilize any destroyed cheddar you like.

The main bit of kitchen gear you have to make these keto chaffles is a waffle creator. I've made chaffles effectively in an ordinary size Belgian waffle producer. What's more, I've made littler size chaffles in a scaled down waffle creator.

Be that as it may, I've had the most achievement utilizing this Dash Mini Waffle Iron to cook chaffles. It is the ideal size to cook them rapidly and make them fresh.

Then, after the chaffle "bread" is prepared, you can fill your sandwich with any fixings you like. For this formula, I've utilized fresh thick-cut bacon and a singed egg. In any case, you can change things up with frankfurter, ham, fried eggs, avocado, hot sauce, and so on. It's truly up to you.

Minor departure from THE CHAFFLE RECIPE

You can add a wide range of flavorings to plain chaffle hitter to make new sorts of chaffles.

Have a go at trying different things with different sorts of cheddar. Cheddar is the first flavor, yet I likewise prefer to utilize Monterrey Jack, Colby, mozzarella cheddar, and so on.

Include flavors, for example, garlic powder, Italian flavoring, Everything But the Bagel flavoring, or grouped herbs.

For a sweet "McGriddle" kind of chaffle, utilize mellow mozzarella cheddar, and include 1 tsp or 2 of sans sugar maple syrup to the hitter.

For considerably lighter chaffles, you can include a teaspoon of coconut flour or a tablespoon of almond flour to the egg blend. For a definitive fluffiest chaffles, include 1/4 tsp preparing powder and a touch of salt.

Fixings

For the chaffles

1 egg

1/2 cup cheddar, destroyed

For the sandwich

2 strips bacon

1 egg

1 cut Cheddar or American cheddar.

Directions

Preheat the waffle creator as per producer directions..

In a little blending bowl, combine egg and destroyed cheddar. Mix until all around consolidated.

Pour one portion of the waffle hitter into the waffle creator. Cook for 3-4 minutes or until brilliant dark colored. Rehash with the second 50% of the hitter.

In a huge dish over medium warmth, cook the bacon until firm, turning varying. Evacuate to deplete on paper towels.

In a similar skillet, in 1 tbsp of saved bacon drippings, fry the egg over medium warmth. Cook until wanted doneness.

Collect the sandwich, and appreciate!

NOTES

If you are utilizing a bigger size waffle producer, you might have the option to cook the entire measure of hitter in one waffle. This will shift with the size of your machine.

SWEEK CINNAMON "SUGAR" CHAFFLE

Cinnamon Roll Chaffles
When I perceived how much everybody adored my Keto Blueberry Chaffle and the Pizza Chaffle I realized I needed to get back in the kitchen and concoct some progressively delicious goodness. I asked my children what the following flavor chaffle ought to be since they are my taste analyzers and they all said something that suggests a flavor like a cinnamon roll.
They love my cinnamon move flapjacks the same amount of as I do and now whenever we make cinnamon move hotcakes or cinnamon move waffles I can appreciate these keto cinnamon move waffles! If you are searching for a low carb cinnamon move waffle that preferences stunning this is it
Supplies expected to make Cinnamon Roll Keto Chaffles
Run Waffle Maker. This thing is AMAZING and you cannot beat the cost! I will have much more keto chaffle plans turning out so you may need to simply get yourself one at this point.
3 little bowls.
Whisk.
Estimating cups
Estimating spoon.
Cinnamon Roll Chaffle Ingredients
1/2 cup destroyed mozzarella cheddar
1 tablespoon almond flour
1 teaspoon cinnamon
1/4 tsp heating powder
1 eggs
1 tsp Granulated Swerve
Cinnamon move twirl Ingredients
1 tbsp margarine
1 tsp cinnamon
2 tsp swerve
Keto Cinnamon Roll Glaze
1 tablespoon margarine

1 tablespoon cream cheddar
1/4 tsp vanilla concentrate
2 tsp swerve confectioners sugar
The most effective method to Make Cinnamon Roll Chaffles
When you are making a chaffle you should utilize a smaller than usual waffle creator with the Dash scaled down waffle producer. Plug in your Mini Dash Waffle producer and let it heat up.
In a little bowl blend the mozzarella cheddar, almond flour, heating powder, egg, cinnamon and swerve. put in a safe spot.
In another little bowl include a tablespoon of margarine, 1 tsp cinnamon, and 2 teaspoons of swerve confectioners sugar. Microwave for 15 seconds and blend well.
Shower the waffle producer with non stick splash and include 1/3 of the hitter to your waffle creator. Twirl in 1/3 of the cinnamon, swerve and margarine blend onto its highest point. Close the waffle producer and let cook for 3-4 minutes.
When the primary cinnamon move chaffle is done, make the second and afterward make the third.
While the third chaffle is cooking place 1 tablespoon margarine and 1 tablespoon of cream cheddar in a little bowl. Warmth in the microwave for 10-15 seconds. Start at 10 and if the cream cheddar isn't sufficiently delicate to blend in with the margarine heat for an extra 5 seconds.
Include the vanilla concentrate and the swerve confectioners sugar to the spread and cream cheddar and blend well utilizing a whisk.
Shower keto cream cheddar coat over chaffle.
Fixings
Cinnamon Roll Chaffle Ingredients
1/2 cup mozzarella cheddar
1 tablespoon almond flour
1/4 tsp heating powder
1 eggs
1 tsp cinnamon
1 tsp Granulated Swerve

Cinnamon move whirl Ingredients
1 tbsp spread
1 tsp cinnamon
2 tsp confectioners swerve
Keto Cinnamon Roll Glaze
1 tablespoon spread
1 tablespoon cream cheddar
1/4 tsp vanilla concentrate
2 tsp swerve confectioners
Directions
Cinnamon Roll Chaffles
Plug in your Mini Dash Waffle creator and let it heat up.

In a little bowl blend the mozzarella cheddar, almond flour, heating powder, egg, 1 teaspoon cinnamon and 1 teaspoon swerve granulated and put in a safe spot.

In another little bowl include a tablespoon of margarine, 1 teaspoon cinnamon, and 2 teaspoons of swerve confectioners' sugar.

Microwave for 15 seconds and blend well.

Shower the waffle producer with nonstick splash and include 1/3 of the hitter to your waffle creator. Whirl in 1/3 of the cinnamon, swerve and margarine blend onto its highest point. Close the waffle creator and let cook for 3-4 minutes.

When the principal cinnamon move chaffle is done, make the second and afterward make the third.

While the third chaffle is cooking place 1 tablespoon spread and 1 tablespoon of cream cheddar in a little bowl. Warmth in the microwave for 10-15 seconds. Start at 10 and if the cream cheddar isn't sufficiently delicate to blend in with the margarine heat for an extra 5 seconds.

Include the vanilla concentrate and the swerve confectioners' sugar to the margarine and cream cheddar and blend well utilizing a whisk.

Sprinkle keto cream cheddar coat over chaffle.

Nourishment

Calories: 180kcal | Carbohydrates: 3g | Protein: 7g | Fat: 16g | Saturated Fat: 9g | Cholesterol: 95mg | Sodium: 221mg | Potassium: 77mg | Fiber: 1g | Sugar: 1g | Vitamin A: 505IU | Calcium: 148mg | Iron: 1mg

Course Breakfast, Dessert, keto, low carb

Cooking American

Catchphrases Cinnamon Roll Chaffle, Keto Cinnamon Roll Chaffle, Keto Cinnamon Roll Waffle

KETO "CINNAMON ROLL" CHAFFLES

Simple, Keto Low-Carb Cinnamon Roll Chaffles is a snappy formula that will tell you the best way to make keto-accommodating waffles utilizing two fixings! Include cinnamon and sugar to get sweet waffles showered with low-carb syrup.

When warmed in a waffle iron, an exquisite waffle is delivered. What's incredible is this strategy will even work for sweet plans. Mozzarella cheddar is about surface. It has next to no flavor. That is the reason your waffles won't have an aftertaste like cheddar! Except if you use enhanced cheddar, similar to cheddar.

The most effective method to MAKE CHAFFLES

Consolidate an egg and 1/2 cup of destroyed mozzarella in a little bowl.

Include vanilla, sugar, and cinnamon.

Mix and add the blend to a lubed waffle dish.

Cook for 2-3 minutes or until the waffle iron demonstrates it has wrapped up.

HOW DO CHAFFLES TASTE?

If you don't improve them, as I would see it, they taste extremely appetizing. I additionally believe that by making them the standard route with simply egg and mozzarella, I taste the egg significantly more.

Appropriately mixing the egg will help counteract this, yet I like the chaffles significantly more with sugar. They will make an incredible substitute for bread and buns in appetizing plans

WHICH WAFFLE IRON TO USE

I would not like to purchase another waffle iron, so I utilized my Belgian waffle producer I have had for a considerable length of time.

Fixings

1 egg

1/2 cup destroyed mozzarella cheddar

1/2 teaspoon vanilla

---

2 tablespoons Zero Calorie Sweetener Use Discount Code: STAYSNATCHED for investment funds

1/2 teaspoon ground cinnamon

Monkfruit Maple Syrup

Guidelines

Add the egg to a bowl and beat. Include the rest of the fixings and blend well.

Plug in the waffle iron and oil the iron with oil or spread.

When hot, include the hitter and close the iron.

I let my waffles cook until the marker light on the iron said they were done. This was around 2 – 2 1/2 minutes. Your planning may shift contingent upon the iron you use.

Cautiously expel the waffle from the iron. I like to utilize a spatula because the waffles are extremely delicate to contact at first.

Let the waffles represent 2-3 minutes. They will solidify.

Notes

Makes 1 enormous waffle or 2 little waffles.

If you are utilizing a scaled down waffle iron, separate the hitter into equal parts to make 2 waffles.

You may have hitter spill out of the waffle iron. This typically transpired if I attempted to uniformly spread the hitter all through the iron myself. Concentrate on spreading it in the iron and not along the edges. When you close the iron the player will round out without anyone else.

I have tried the formula utilizing granular sugar and Confectioner's Sweetener. Both worked fine.

If you don't improve chaffles, as I would like to think, they taste extremely exquisite. I likewise imagine that by making them the standard path with simply egg and mozzarella, I taste the egg significantly more.

I tried the formula utilizing 1 tablespoon of sugar, and felt like the chaffles tasted eggy. Don't hesitate to change in accordance with your taste and inclination.

You can freeze the chaffles. They may soften when you defrost. You can have a go at crisping them in a toaster.

SWEET AND SAVORY MILKY CHAFFLE

You folks, evidently, I have been living in the waffle dull ages, because, chaffles are extremely popular right now in Keto land and if you have no clue what a chaffle is, you are in for a delectable shock . This may simply be life changing, or if nothing else keto lifestyle modifying as the cherished chaffle is a low carb nourishment that will take your keto plans to a totally different measurement. From what I comprehend, the word chaffle is a cross breed of cheddar and waffle... .Tada, chaffle.

All that's needed is two fixings, can be made in only minutes, and is excessively a good time for releasing significant innovativeness!

My sister originally cautioned me to this new pattern, and gifted me with a smaller than usual scramble waffle producer. You can make this in a full size iron, however the small scale is extremely fun, and very reasonable.

A couple of tips I have adapted up until this point:

1) Thinly cut cheddar is extremely useful. I truly like the Sargento brand.

2) The less egg you use, the crispier chaffle you will accomplish

3) seasonings can be supernatural (we truly appreciate bagel flavoring)

As a last note... ..nutty spread on a sweet chaffle is next level, if you're missing dearest PB&J's from adolescence (or peanut spread and nectar for my situation) this truly hits the spot!

Gear

smaller than normal waffle iron

ordinary waffle iron

Fixings

1 egg

4 cuts cheddar Thinly cut

3 cuts Bacon Cooked

1 lettuce leaf

2 cuts tomato

---

2 tbsp mayonnaise

Directions

Take 1 egg and break and mix in an estimating cup. Utilizing an estimating cup makes it simpler to pour and utilize the egg.

Oil your little waffle iron with a keto well-disposed cooking shower (we utilized avocado splash)

Let waffle iron warmth up

Take two cuts of cheddar and cut corners off (Optional) this encourages it fit into a small scale waffle producer. Skip if utilizing a full estimated waffle creator.

Cautiously place cheddar on hot waffle surface.

Let cheddar start to liquefy

As cheddar dissolves pour a limited quantity of your beat eggs over the softening cheddar.

Then include a second cut of cheddar over the layer of cheddar and egg that is as of now cooking.

Cautiously close your waffle iron and let cook for around 3 minutes

Following 3 minutes your Chaffle ought to be fresh and you can cautiously evacuate it.

Rehash Steps above to make a second Chaffle.

While your second Chaffle is cooking. Include mayonnaise, Tomato, lettuce and bacon to your first Chaffle cut to start assembling your Chaffle BLT.

After your second Chaffle is done cooking, include mayo and make the most of your Keto Chaffle BLT!

Notes

3 - 4 Net Carbs for the BLT. A large portion of these carbs are from the lettuce and tomato.

We gauge for the 2 chaffles without the meat, veggies and sauces would approach = 1 net carb.

Sustenance

Serving: 4oz | Calories: 699kcal | Carbohydrates: 5g | Protein: 20g | Fat: 65g | Saturated Fat: 20g | Cholesterol: 219mg | Sodium: 684mg | Potassium: 366mg | Fiber: 1g | Sugar: 2g | Vitamin A: 2464IU | Vitamin C: 12mg | Calcium: 25mg | Iron: 1mg

CPSIA information can be obtained
at www.ICGtesting.com
Printed in the USA
LVHW082048180121
676770LV00001B/10

9 781801 601207